More Praise for
Surviving Our Catastrophes

"If the human race can look back without despair on what it did to itself in the twentieth century (and may well be about to do again), then we should thank the unflinching wisdom of Robert Jay Lifton. This short, utterly necessary book is written at the climax of a very long life, by a man who has looked straight into the black sun of Auschwitz and Hiroshima and yet preserved his moral eyesight. . . . Lifton writes here about victims who become survivors . . . of catastrophes present and to come: Covid-19, nuclear threat, climate change. We have to learn from the survivors of catastrophe 'if we are to learn the truth about ourselves, if we are to go on living as a species.'"

—Neal Ascherson, Scottish journalist and author of
Black Sea and the novel *The Death of the Fronsac*

"Lifton escorts us on a soul-searching journey and gives us an emotional and intellectual road map for accepting and living through catastrophes using what he calls 'survivor power.' This book is not just a captivating read; it's also a life-affirming experience."

—Dr. Michael Osterholm, Regents Professor,
McKnight Presidential Endowed Chair in Public Health,
University of Minnesota, and former Science Envoy for
Health Security on behalf of the U.S. Department of State

"Lifton, more than anyone alive today, can serve as a wise and lucid guide . . . [to] the remarkably life-affirming responses of survivors of atrocities, and the larger human capacity for collective renewal."

—Bessel Van Der Kolk, author of *The Body Keeps the Score*

"With the same intellectual rigor and passionate commitment he has brought to his life's work, Robert Jay Lifton explains how the way we process and memorialize catastrophe—Hiroshima, the AIDS plague, the murderous early days of the Covid pandemic—can reveal, and mobilize, what he calls our 'human commonality.' It's a book we can all be grateful for."

—Daniel Okrent, author of *The Guarded Gate* and *Last Call*

"This exquisite distillation of a genius-life's wisdom turns our age of troubles into a time of unexpected affirmation and abundant possibility. Robert Jay Lifton's briefest book is—stunningly—his magnum opus."

—James Carroll, author of *The Truth at the Heart of the Lie*

"Lifton offers a powerful and clear physical and spiritual road map of how to navigate our pain after a personal or global disaster: see it, feel it, own it, share it, and use it."

—Sohaila Abdulali, author of *What We Talk About When We Talk About Rape*

Also by Robert Jay Lifton

Thought Reform and the Psychology of Totalism:
A Study of "Brainwashing" in China (1961)

Death in Life: Survivors of Hiroshima (1968)

Home from the War: Vietnam Veterans—
Neither Victims Nor Executioners (1973)

The Broken Connection: On Death and the Continuity of Life (1979)

The Nazi Doctors: Medical Killing and the Psychology of Genocide
(1986)

The Genocidal Mentality: Nazi Holocaust and Nuclear Threat
(with Eric Markusen) (1990)

The Protean Self: Human Resilience in an Age of Fragmentation
(1993)

Hiroshima in America: Fifty Years of Denial
(with Greg Mitchell) (1995)

Destroying the World to Save It: Aum Shinrikyō, Apocalyptic Violence,
and the New Global Terrorism (1999)

Witness to an Extreme Century: A Memoir (2011)

The Climate Swerve: Reflections on Mind, Hope, and Survival (2017)

Losing Reality: On Cults, Cultism, and the Mindset of Political and
Religious Zealotry (2019)

SURVIVING OUR CATASTROPHES

Resilience and Renewal from Hiroshima
to the Covid-19 Pandemic

ROBERT JAY LIFTON

THE
NEW
PRESS

NEW YORK
LONDON

"A Psychiatrist in the World" will appear in slightly different form in the collection
Driven to Write: 39 Authors on the Mysteries of Their Art and Craft, edited by Michael
Slevin and Ellen Pinksy (forthcoming).

Requests for permission to reproduce selections from this book should be made through
our website: https://thenewpress.com/contact.

Published in the United States by The New Press, New York, 2023
Distributed by Two Rivers Distribution

ISBN 978-1-62097-815-3 (hc)
ISBN 978-1-62097-829-0 (ebook)
CIP data is available

The New Press publishes books that promote and enrich public discussion and
understanding of the issues vital to our democracy and to a more equitable world. These
books are made possible by the enthusiasm of our readers; the support of a committed
group of donors, large and small; the collaboration of our many partners in the
independent media and the not-for-profit sector; booksellers, who often hand-sell New
Press books; librarians; and above all by our authors.

www.thenewpress.com

Book design and composition by Bookbright Media
This book was set in Adobe Garamond and Bodoni 72
Printed in the United States of America

2 4 6 8 10 9 7 5 3 1

For survivors who witness catastrophe
and bring us hope.

Everything is possible in history.

—José Ortega y Gasset

For the real question is whether the "brighter future" is really always so distant. What if, on the contrary, it has been here for a long time already, and only our blindness and weakness has prevented us from seeing it around us and within us, and kept us from developing it?

—Václav Havel

Contents

A Psychiatrist in the World

For me, to be active in the world means to write about it. But to explain how I became a writer I must tell a story.

My story begins with a walk in Hong Kong in late April of 1954, when I was twenty-eight years old. I wandered through the crowded colonial streets past small Chinese noodle stands and elegant European dress stores, but my mind was on neither the people nor the streets. I was painfully preoccupied with an important life decision I was trying to make.

I had been living in Hong Kong, together with my wife, BJ, for about three months, staying in a garret hotel room that we somehow found comfortable. I had been interviewing both Westerners and Chinese who had been subjected on the mainland to a remarkable process called "thought reform" (or, more loosely, "brainwashing"). The process was always coercive in its use of criticism, self-criticism, and confession. But it also called forth powerful exhortation on behalf of a new Chinese dawn, seeking to bring about a change in identity from the Confucian filial son or daughter to the filial Communist (or Maoist), and to do so in hundreds of millions of people. With Westerners, mostly missionaries, "reeducated" in prison, there could be considerable violence used to extract false confessions of secret espionage.

Hong Kong was supposed to have been just a stop on a leisurely round-the-world trip that began in Japan, where I had arranged to be discharged from the military after two years of service as an Air Force psychiatrist.

I had joined the military only because I had been subjected to a "doctor draft" and sent to Japan and then to Taegu in Korea, though never close to a combat area. I became fascinated by East Asia and its extraordinary postwar directions.

My final military assignment was to interview repatriated American prisoners of war released from Chinese captivity in North Korea. The interviews were done first in the South Korean port city of Incheon, just below the thirty-eighth parallel and the no-man's-land dividing the two Koreas, and then on a troopship called the *General Pope* on a fifteen-day voyage from Incheon to San Francisco. The repatriated POWs had been subjected to an export version of thought reform, and the military environment imposed constraints on my encounters with them.

Mainland China was then mostly cut off from the Western world, and in Hong Kong I met "China watchers"—scholars, diplomats, and teachers, who were European, American, and Chinese—with whom I had lively discussions about the appeal and excesses of the Communist revolution. They in turn were eager to hear my impressions, as a psychiatrist, of a thought-reform process they found confusing. They put me in touch with Chinese students and intellectuals, as well as Western missionaries and teachers, who agreed to be interviewed about the psychology of the process they had experienced. I was immersed in a powerful historical moment and experienced both fascination and a sense of adventure.

But I also felt uneasy at being isolated from American institutions, from the serious business of psychiatric and psychoanalytic training and the proper pursuit of my professional career—that is, removed from the structures of real life. Besides, our money was running out.

I was very reluctant to leave Hong Kong but could not seem to imagine staying. BJ was game either way. Hence my solitary walk.

My conflict was played out by first making a "decision" that we could not stay in Hong Kong, and then within a day reversing that decision by submitting an application for a research grant that would enable us to do just that.

I would later comment that the military saved me from a conventional life and I have never shown it much gratitude. A friend of mine put things differently: "You did not make the decision, the decision made you." (Unsurprisingly, that friend is a Zen Buddhist.)

The decision made me a writer. Not consciously—the words "writer" and "writing" did not enter my conflicted inner dialogue. What did concern me was whether I could become a *psychiatrist in the world*, a vague but compelling image that contrasted favorably with one of spending most of my professional life in a comfortable New York therapy office.

In fact I had already published a paper for the *American Journal of Psychiatry* about my interviews with returning prisoners of war. I was discovering, as others have, that no exploration of an event is complete—for others or oneself—until one writes about it, or at least puts it into some kind of mental structure.

In my case everything started with being a *listening writer*, with interviews that enabled me to take in the words of someone else as the basis for what I would write. Such listening came to anchor my work in general, whether with those Chinese or Westerners who had been "reeducated," Hiroshima survivors, Vietnam veterans, or Nazi doctors. In those interviews I encouraged a back-and-forth that was much more of a dialogue than was any form of conventional psychiatric exchange. At the same time I kept what I called a "research diary," dictated immediately after the interview and making use of written notes I had made (mostly quotations from the interviewee). When I later organized my findings, I referred more to this research diary than to the unwieldy tape recordings, though the latter were invaluable for checking on actual words expressed during the interview.

I was also, as I came to realize, a *witnessing writer*. I was aware of having unusual access to a process that was profound and troubling, and I wanted to retell it accurately and make it known, that is, to bear witness to what I was learning. That meant taking a stand and becoming an advocate, combining scholarship and activism. That combination has been crucial to me throughout my work.

My writing itself became a form of activism. In that

process my dictation did not stop with the research diary but extended to my overall presentation of my observations and interpretations. With thought reform and all other subsequent work, I have been a *talking writer*. Rather than the hand-brain interactions of most writers typing their work or even writing by hand, mine has been a brain-larynx connection. Even when I compose a blurb for a book or work on a short paragraph of any kind, I do so by speaking it into my Dictaphone, utilizing this old-fashioned instrument because it is more malleable than digital counterparts for quick shifts in spoken words. In all this, the computer screen is of importance only to enable me to visualize what I have spoken in order to redictate subsequent drafts until I am satisfied with the words on the screen.

Friends have told me that this auditory method makes my writing more "conversational," which is true enough, but there is more to it. Whether listening or speaking, I almost instantly merge the auditory with the visual: what I heard from Hiroshima survivors enabled me to see immediately before me the terrible scenes of death and pain they described. It is possible that in some way my auditory emphasis gave special intensity to its visual translation.

This admittedly idiosyncratic method seems to feed

my psychological and historical—that is, psychohistorical
—imagination.

There is also an important factor of place and space. My sequence has been to obtain my verbal information out in "the field," whether that be Hong Kong or Hiroshima or Germany or some other country in Europe or Asia— though with Vietnam veterans the "field" was the United States.

I have then come "home" to my study, a place for me of isolation and reimagining, wherever that study may be. My "mother of all studies" has been a separate renovated shack, with a glimpse of the ocean, adjoining my Wellfleet house, where I have been able to place thick folders of tran- scribed interview recordings and research diaries on solid oak tables to carry through my version of sorting and writ- ing. But I have had smaller replicas of that study in other places, such as New Haven, New York, or Cambridge, depending on which university I was affiliated with at the time. My study came to take on the character of a special space where, with considerable difficulty, I might find the words I need.

In some traditions it is held that scholarship and activ- ism must remain entirely separate, and ne'er the twain shall meet. I think the opposite is true. Scholarship is rendered meaningful by activism, and activism is significantly informed by scholarship. Both need to be undertaken with discipline.

Preface

A book completed just after the author's ninety-sixth birthday has to have a history of its own. That includes nearly seventy years of probing the psychological and historical impact of holocaust, mass violence, and renewal. Of bearing witness to and confronting as a psychiatrist, writer, and activist the catastrophes of the twentieth and twenty-first centuries.

When my daughter was a young girl, she once asked me why I studied such terrible things instead of more pleasant ones. My answer at the time was vague and probably unconvincing to both of us, but I think I have a better answer now, many decades later. It is that one must examine a society's response to catastrophe in order to have any sense of that society's resilience and health. Such work is an act of resistance and always implies an alternative to catastrophe.

These days Americans are confronting all too much catastrophe: climate and nuclear threats; the war in Ukraine; the attack from within on our democratic procedures—including the peaceful transfer of power after a presidential election; and the pervasive immediate catastrophe of the Covid-19 pandemic.

Like everyone else in early 2020, I had no idea how

much my life would be changed by Covid-19. By late February, my partner, Nancy Rosenblum, and I had begun to experience the general fear that was building in New York City—concern about catching the virus by pushing elevator buttons, feeling uncomfortable when tenants from other floors got on, wondering if we should wash our grocery cans. We were worried when Governor Cuomo announced the first Covid case in New York State on March 1 and the first death on March 10. My son, who followed the issue closely, urged us to leave the city for a less populated area.

I was in my nineties and Nancy in her seventies, so we were at considerable risk. We took advantage of roots we had on outer Cape Cod, where we first met, and of homes there in which we were used to living half the year. We were aware of our privileged status in having that option.

We left in mid-March, just before the New York lockdown, as Covid cases in the state climbed past five thousand, including more than forty deaths. Yet, as we passed the Wellfleet cinema on Route 6, we were sufficiently innocent of any understanding of how the virus spread to wonder whether there would be a decent film playing there that weekend and were surprised to find that the cinema was closed.

For the following year and a half, like many others throughout the world, we greatly restricted in-person visits of family and friends. And although that has changed somewhat with the development of Covid vaccines, our lives remain considerably altered by a virus that continues to stalk us.

We settled into the Cape, and after a few months gave up our apartment in New York. That entailed elaborate arrangements for storing our possessions, all the more so because they were made at a distance. I had the feeling that much of my life went into storage together with the books and papers, paintings, and clothes. Nancy and I continue to have many talks about our future, about the uncertainties of when and whether we would feel safe to return to New York.

In January 2021, the incoming Biden administration brought reason and science to the struggle against Covid, in contrast to Trump's deadly irresponsibility. Even so, government agencies remained less than fully clear in their recommendations about masks and distancing. Nancy and I were caught up in the larger national and world conflict between powerfully contradictory impulses: toward caution and restraint in connection with the pandemic as opposed to opening up the society and returning to something like normal function.

The catastrophes that face America and the world are daunting, and there is no single approach or individual mind that can fully encompass them. But while living in relative isolation and continuing with my work, I realized that I could have something to say based on what I have learned from studies I have done—on Chinese Communist "thought reform," the atomic bombing of Hiroshima, antiwar Vietnam veterans, Nazi doctors, "climate swerve" (recognition of climate truths), and resistance to the reality of Covid-19 and to the vaccines that have been so important for controlling its spread.

Much of my work has centered on what we generally speak of as mass trauma—on pain inflicted on the bodies and minds of large groups of people. But I have focused less on trauma per se than on the experience of the survivor. The survivor suffers from catastrophe but can also be crucial to overcoming it. By looking closely at the struggles of survivors, we can learn much about catastrophe itself and about the larger human capacity for collective renewal. And that is what this book is about.

My work in Hiroshima was a key turning point for me.

Before that, under the influence of Erik Erikson, I had focused on issues of identity and identity change. But in Hiroshima I encountered a death-saturated environment, the understanding of which required me to seek a model or paradigm that emphasized the continuity of life and at the same time gave death its due.

I thought of Sigmund Freud, who had experienced the death-saturated environment of World War I and tried to make sense of the widespread slaughter he had witnessed. But the only place he could find for it in his conceptual structure was the death drive. This sweeping instinctual vision has confused psychological thought ever since. I reread Freud through the lens of my Hiroshima experience. I translated his focus on instinct into a focus on the way we symbolize life and death. The book I later wrote, *The Broken Connection*, explored the place of death in the continuity of life.

I hadn't probed the issue of death and death symbolism until my Hiroshima study. Rather than becoming antinuclear because of that study, I would say that I went to Hiroshima because I was antinuclear. The activist tail was wagging the scholarly dog. I had been exposed to a group called the Committee of Correspondence in Cambridge,

Massachusetts, led by David Riesman in the late 1950s. Riesman was an early antinuclear academic, a sociologist who made use of his professional knowledge to probe ways in which nuclear weapons were harming our society and our institutions. I wished to become, as a psychiatrist, a similarly involved professional. So when I was in Japan in the early 1960s to do a study of Japanese youth, I decided to pay a visit to Hiroshima.

I was stunned to discover that, despite the tragic turning point in human history that had occurred with the dropping of the bomb on that city, no one had done a comprehensive study of what happened there. I was able to convince the head of my department at Yale, where I had been given a research chair, of the importance of the kind of study I could perform in Hiroshima.

I tried to do the work systematically by means of modified psychoanalytic interviews that lent themselves to exchange and dialogue. The book I wrote about the study, *Death in Life: Survivors of Hiroshima*, was my scholarly contribution to antinuclear activism.

Now as we encounter renewed talk of the use of nuclear weapons, with mention of possible nuclear Armageddon, I am haunted by what I learned of a "tiny" nuclear weapon by present standards. In Hiroshima that lesson was: one plane, one bomb, one city.

The six months I spent in Hiroshima interviewing survivors of the atomic bomb were life changing both personally and professionally. It was there that I became aware that we human beings, with our escalated conflicts, were capable of destroying our entire species, and possibly the entire planet. But I also learned from that study that survivors of the most extreme catastrophe could take on collective efforts toward reestablishing the flow of life.

The experience of Hiroshima survivors became so important to my study that I included in my book a detailed exploration of the phenomenon of the survivor of trauma of any kind. This was the beginning of my preoccupation with survivors. They were thrust into prominence by the catastrophes of the twentieth century, and they turn out to be crucial to our recovery from catastrophe in general.

The veterans I later interviewed as survivors of the Vietnam War also left a profound impression on me. From them I learned that ordinary people, no better or worse than you or me, could, under certain aggressive military policies and resulting psychological conditions, all too readily engage in mass slaughter and the mutilation of bodies. That is, they could become part of an *atrocity-producing situation*.

I also learned that some of those American survivors of Vietnam were capable of change that could be fairly rapid and impressively lasting, of looking critically at their behavior and altering their earlier view of the war, their relationships to others, their family life, and their own violent tendencies. That observation called into question much that psychological professionals have long believed about the limits to individual and collective change. I found that significant change can begin with confronting one's death encounter, raising questions about dying and killing.

It also became clear to me over time that, although the Vietnam War was notorious for its overall atrocity-producing situation, all wars are catastrophes in which such murderous environments exist. But so does the capacity for men and women to undergo life-enhancing change.

In my work on Nazi doctors I was confronted with the ultimate evil of a murderously planned catastrophe of unprecedented dimensions. I was struck by the central role in the killing by members of my own medical profession, particularly the mass murder of Jews, but also of other groups considered "life unworthy of life." In the work I focused on the Nazi principle of *killing to heal*, the need to kill millions of Jews to "heal" the "Nordic race." I called this reversal of healing and killing the *medicalization of killing*.

Yet in the killing factory of Auschwitz I also encountered physicians who, as prisoners themselves, somehow managed to sustain a healing ethos, though they had almost nothing in the way of medication to offer other than a few aspirins. Those former prisoner-doctors were mostly Jews but could also be non-Jewish Poles or Germans, who made consistent efforts to save lives. I understood that these prisoner-doctors were survivors who had a unique capacity to witness the Nazi medicalized killing.

When I interviewed Jewish former prisoner-doctors, I could not help identifying with them and contrasting their experience with my own comfortable life in America. I was perhaps ten years younger than most of them, but similar in coming from a middle-class Jewish family that placed great value on a medical education. Only a few twists in history protected me from an ordeal such as theirs or worse.

Whatever anti-Semitism I experienced as a child or young adult did not prevent me from pursuing an idiosyncratic career in which I have been a frequent critic of the

American political status quo. I came to speak of aspects of this status quo as a *malignant normality*, in which destructive behavior could be routinized and accepted as part of the social landscape. My activism has not led to my being silenced or persecuted; it has mostly been respected and sometimes honored.

People often ask me how I can be "courageous" or "strong" enough to take in the collective horrors I describe. My answer is that it is more a question of finding a balance in my work about how much I am able to *feel*. I need to take in some of the pain the work uncovers but at the same time create a measure of professional distance, something on the order of a surgeon performing a delicate operation or a clinical psychiatrist carrying out an interview with a depressed patient.

I remember a moment of exchange I had with the Auschwitz survivor Elie Wiesel. I told him how my early work with Nazi doctors was causing me to have nightmares in which I was surrounded by dying people behind barbed wire, and my wife and children were there as well. He looked at me steadily and said quietly, "Good. Now you can do the study." He meant that I was sufficiently open to the Auschwitz experience to be able to study it. But he also knew that I had to find a way to limit the pain I experienced in order to be an accurate researcher.

Along the way I have developed an identity of one who does this kind of demanding research, and holding on to that identity enables me to feel that it is appropriate for me, as a psychiatric investigator, to continue to do the work. I also experience a sense of satisfaction having to do with my staying power in getting that work done and making it widely available.

I have required a certain amount of self-protection, of what is sometimes called care of the self. That has entailed limiting my daily exposure to the painful details of the work and spending considerable time in a separate world of reading books and seeing films of a different order. That separate world must include considerable love. For me, it has also included passionate rooting for my favorite baseball team, the Los Angeles Dodgers, because they were so important to me as a child in Brooklyn before they moved to the West Coast.

I have frequently told friends and students that I have a policy of "not reading or working on that [catastrophic] stuff after nine p.m.," advising them to do the same should they embark on such studies.

I also have what can be called an avocation, which takes the form of drawing bird cartoons, and have published them in two books, one called *Birds* and the other *Psychobirds*. These creatures enable me to bring humor, mostly gallows humor, to catastrophe. I have no artistic talent—the birds are stick figures—but they can say things in very different ways from my other work. The example I include here deals with nuclear holocaust. One bird says, "Do your studies demonstrate that American society can recover from a nuclear attack?" And the other answers, "Yes! All except the people."

Those actually caught up in disaster can express their own gallows humor. For instance, a man I interviewed in Hiroshima who was the owner of a crematorium told me that, when experiencing the bomb, he thought it very convenient that he was so close to his crematorium.

But whatever protective steps I take, there is no avoiding —nor do I want to avoid—a certain degree of immersion into destructiveness and evil that threatens my own sense of self. Such an immersion is the only path to deepened knowledge of these events, and to the re-creation of self and world.

The core issues of this book, having to do with catastrophe and survivors, are at the center of my work. I have found that survivors can possess certain kinds of wisdom and influence, can be a reminder of pain, possibility, and hope.

The emergence of Covid-19 survivor groups who demand a hearing has great significance. Those survivor groups have been concerned both with the nature of the virus, particularly of long Covid, and also with ways of improving our society's capacity to cope with it. They press us toward a species-wide ethic, quite beyond that of immediate Covid concerns.

I say all this as a third-generation Jewish American sensitive to the saturation with death of the last half of the twentieth century and the beginning of the twenty-first. My goal, wherever possible, has been to combine witness with illumination. I labor to understand where we are, how we got here, and what we might do collectively to survive.

Surviving Our Catastrophes

1

Catastrophe and Survivors

Catastrophes are always with us. There is a large historical—one might even say evolutionary—flow, from relatively stable structures, to the social breakdown that comes with catastrophe, to survivors' efforts at renewal.

Such catastrophes include wars, nuclear attacks, Auschwitz-style killing factories, earthquakes, droughts, uncontrollable fires, widespread flooding, and lethal pandemics. While some of these catastrophes are spoken of as "natural," all of them have a crucial human contribution, so much so that there is reason to doubt the existence of any purely natural catastrophe. Whatever the catastrophe, survivors can become a crucial force for reconstituting their society.

I am making two assumptions here. First, that a society must recognize the reality of a catastrophe in order to cope with it. And second, that survivors are powerful agents in this process.

What, then, is a survivor? A survivor is someone who has been confronted with death in some bodily or psychic fashion and has himself or herself remained alive. I have come to view survivors as a special group with particular psychological characteristics. But in order to experience oneself as a survivor, one must overcome the sense of being an incapacitated victim.

The word "victim," derived from the Latin *victima*, had the late-fifteenth-century meaning of a living creature being offered as a "sacrifice to a supernatural power." In subsequent centuries it came to mean a "person who was hurt, tortured, or killed by another," or "made to suffer . . . from disease or disaster"; and still later, a "person taken advantage of . . . cheated or duped."

To be a victim, then, is to be helpless, to be acted upon by others for their own purposes, to be harmed, deceived, even destroyed. A victim can feel immobilized psychically as well as physically, preoccupied mainly with his or her misfortune.

The word "survivor," in contrast, derives from the late Latin *supervīvĕre*—*vīvĕre* meaning "to live" and *super* suggesting "over" or "beyond." So the word came to mean "to continue to live on after the death of another," or "after the end of some condition or occurrence . . . to remain alive, to live on."

A survivor, then, is an active agent of the continuation of life.

There is always a paradox in connection with the survivor. The word suggests an encounter with death, and in that way puts death at the center of trauma. But survivor also means remaining alive, whatever the threat or assault.

Survivors of any catastrophe experience a *death imprint*, a lasting image of people dying in that disaster. That death imprint can quickly bring about a cessation of feeling, a form of *psychic numbing*, as a way of protecting the mind from an otherwise unmanageable and self-shattering form of death anxiety. In extreme catastrophes, the death imprint can be associated with a breakdown of faith in the function of the larger human matrix.

We humans are meaning-hungry creatures, and survivors are particularly *starved for meaning* that can help them "explain" their ordeal. Only by finding such meaning can they tell their story and begin to cope with grief and loss.

Survivors are mourners, and their negotiation of the mourning process is crucial both to their renewed energies and to the potential wisdom they may acquire from their death immersion. Survivors may connect the meaning they achieve with a *survivor mission*, and some of them may devote much of their lives to combatting the catastrophe they had undergone.

That mission can be personal: if my brother dies of

prostate cancer, I may become involved in raising money or otherwise contributing to the treatment of that disease. Or it may be collective: if my city has been destroyed by an atomic bomb, I may join with others in telling the world about that catastrophe and in advocating for the abolition of nuclear weapons.

There are always two possibilities for anyone encountering death: closing down or opening out. When we close down, our pain becomes isolated and unapproachable. When we can open out, we may connect with others and can even become part of a remarkable group who have known grotesque versions of dying and yet returned to the living. In that way survivors can call forth the transformative power of the death encounter. But survivors are never entirely free of the struggle between closing down and opening out.

Leaders in a post-catastrophe environment can sense the importance of survivor agency. For instance, decades after the dropping of the bomb in Hiroshima, one prominent figure there expressed to me his concern about the degree of "victim consciousness" and the need to actively overcome it in order to contribute to the city's and the world's renewal. He was suggesting that survivors are engaged in a continuous effort to transcend their victimization.

Both collective and individual mourning can be impaired by the very dimensions of a catastrophe—by the vastness and confusion of killing and dying and the absence of bodies or knowledge of particular deaths, as was the case in Auschwitz and Hiroshima. Even when mourning is impaired in this way, survivors can diminish their grief by collectively bearing witness to what they have experienced and by becoming part of groups that tell the world what they have been through.

That shift from victim consciousness into the ethos of the survivor can be enhanced by "emergent leaders," usually themselves survivors who unexpectedly appear from outside official structures. These leaders may rally other survivors into significant group efforts that contribute to healing. Members of such groups experience solidarity, find mutual support, and express their pain while beginning to recognize themselves as active survivors.

There are always distinctions among survivors in regard to their death encounter, as we have observed in our Covid pandemic. The pandemic envelops the world and can cause death anxiety in everyone. There are those who personally experience serious versions of the disease, including long Covid, or have family members or close friends who suffer or die from it. They are the haunted survivors whose experience with the illness immerses them in death. But the rest of us, who have milder cases or do not contract the disease at all, are also survivors—less consumed by death anxiety yet never free of it.

Significant survivor expression in connection with the Covid pandemic has occurred. Groups have taken shape, with names like Survivor Corps, Covid Survivors for Change, Marked by Covid, and Young Widows and Widowers of Covid-19. Such groups can combine knowledge from patients and scientists in their insistence on learning more about the pandemic, knowledge that could serve not only themselves but the larger society.

How does the knowledge that we are all survivors of Covid affect our behavior? It could be a step toward channeling the much broader sense of death anxiety in the direction of potential action. Grief and pain, when shared, can become seeds of activism.

2

The Prophetic Survivors
of Hiroshima

The atomic bombing of Hiroshima in 1945 provides a special kind of illumination for our present struggles with the Covid-19 pandemic—both in its catastrophic destructiveness and in the significance of its survivors.

I arrived in Hiroshima for the first time in 1962, a thirty-six-year-old psychiatric researcher. What I learned there has affected everything I have felt or done since.

Hiroshima survivors were subjected to the most extreme kind of death encounter, from which they emerged to become the center of peace movements in their city and throughout the world.

I had intended a brief visit. But very quickly I became aware that the overall impact of this revolutionary weapon had not been studied. There had been research on the physical aftereffects of the bomb, and there had been brief commentaries here and there on the behavior of some of the survivors at the time of the bomb and afterward. But there had been no systematic examination of the entire catastrophe, of the individual-psychological and collective historical impact of the bomb.

That neglect of research on Hiroshima had much to do with the pain involved—the deeply upsetting images to which an investigator had to be exposed. Research was also sidelined in the early years by victims' need for help rather than study.

Nobody really knows how many people were killed in Hiroshima. Variously estimated from 63,000 to 240,000 or more, the official figure is usually given as 78,000, but the city of Hiroshima estimates 200,000—the total encompassing between 25 and 50 percent of the city's then daytime population. This enormous disparity is related to the extreme confusion at the time, to differing methods of calculation, and to underlying emotional influences—quite apart from mathematical considerations—which have at times affected the estimators. An accurate estimate may never be possible, but what can be said is that *all of Hiroshima immediately became involved in the atomic catastrophe.*

The term *hibakusha* (explosion-affected person[s]), when used for atomic bomb survivors, suggests a little more than merely having encountered the bomb and a little less than having experienced definite injury from it. The category of hibakusha, according to the official definition, includes four groups of people considered to have had significant amounts of radiation exposure: those who at the time of the bomb were within the city limits, those who came into the city within fourteen days of the bombing, those who had various kinds of physical contact with bomb victims, and those who were in utero at the time and whose mothers fit into any of the first three groups.

I too had initially avoided the city and can attest to the great anxiety and pain I came to experience there, so great that for a short period of time I doubted whether I would be able to continue with the study. But that anxiety diminished sufficiently for me to carry out my professional function of interview research over the rest of my half year in Hiroshima.

In those interviews, hibakusha attempted to describe what they found indescribable: the extremity of victimization from which they had to emerge to become survivors and tell their story. They conveyed to me a fear of *invisible contamination*, the sense of a weapon that not only kills and destroys on a colossal scale but also leaves behind in the bodies of those exposed to it a deadly poison that may emerge at any time and strike down its victims.

A history professor described to me how, soon after the bomb, he looked down at the city from a high suburb and saw that: "Hiroshima had disappeared. . . . I was shocked by the sight. . . . Hiroshima didn't exist—that was mainly what I saw—Hiroshima just didn't exist."

In a similar vein, a prominent Japanese physician, himself injured by the bomb, wrote that he could not find
words for what he witnessed: "I had to revise my meaning
of the word destruction . . . devastation may be a better
word, but really I know of no word or words to describe the
view from my twisted iron hospital bed."

His difficulty with words, his sense of the inadequacy of
the words "destruction" and "devastation," had to do with
the extent of the bomb's annihilation: the sea of death at
the time it fell, and its unique and lethal radiation effects.
From a split-second exposure to the weapon, one experienced a permanent encounter with death, not just death
but grotesque and mysterious forms of death.

A well-known writer, herself a hibakusha, was struck by
how "our surroundings changed so greatly in one instant,"
and told of "a fearful silence, which made me feel that all
people . . . were dead." Other hibakusha described themselves to me as having been "walking ghosts"; or, as one
man put it, "I was not really alive."

Hours after the bomb fell, people began to experience a
dreadful fear of invisible contamination. They had bizarre
combinations of symptoms including severe diarrhea and
weakness, bleeding from all the body orifices and into the

skin—the dreaded "purple spots"—high fever, extremely low white blood cell counts (when such studies could be done), loss of body hair, and often a progressive course until death. Ordinary people spoke of a mysterious "poison," and doctors initially suspected some kind of epidemic disease.

Rumors that quickly spread among hibakusha held not only that everyone in Hiroshima would be dead within months or years, but that trees, grass, and flowers would never again grow in Hiroshima; from that day on, the city would be unable to sustain vegetation of any kind. The meaning here was that nature was drying up altogether, life was being extinguished at its source—an ultimate form of desolation that not only encompassed human death but went beyond it.

Within a few years after the bomb fell, doctors discovered an increase in different forms of leukemia among hibakusha, and over decades there have been increases in various forms of cancer—first thyroid cancer, and then cancer of the breast, lung, stomach, bone marrow, and other areas.

Nor did the impact end with one's own body or life. There was the fear that this invisible contamination would manifest itself in the next generation, because it is known that such abnormalities *can* be caused by radiation. As a knowledgeable survivor put it during one of my return visits to Hiroshima: "Well, maybe the next generation is okay after all, but what about the third generation?" There is no end point for perceived damage, or for anxiety.

Hibakusha underwent what can be called a second victimization in the form of significant discrimination in two fundamental areas of life: marriage and work. The "logic" of the discrimination was that survivors were undesirable for marriage because they might have unhealthy children; they were unsuitable for jobs because they could be physically incapable of steady work. But the deeper, often unconscious feeling about atomic bomb survivors was that they were death-tainted, reminders of a fearful event people did not want to be reminded of, that they were carriers, so to speak, of the dreaded "A-bomb disease."

Yet that same hibakusha experience could take on added importance when it came to be associated with what was called "social significance," with making a special contribution to knowledge of and opposition to nuclear weapons. Certain hibakusha became emergent leaders who could mobilize their own conflict and pain to make psychological contact with the experience of hibakusha in general, and seek public action on behalf of the larger group.

One such man was a low-ranking city official who, in the days and months following the bombing, took over from ineffectual superiors in a fierce personal crusade to keep people alive, finding food and clothing and organizing cooperative efforts. He brought to those efforts energy and ingenuity that was both intuitive and transcendent: "I did not know I was doing this, as I was working like a man in a dream. . . . For a year . . . I simply was not aware of whether I was living or not."

Intrinsic to his leadership was his personal fear. He was "terrified" by his low white blood cell counts and suspicious symptoms of invisible contamination. He was also deeply conflicted about neglecting family members in favor of his larger crusade. Unlike some other emergent leaders, he did not recede from public life but remained a prominent figure whose skills could become institutionalized on behalf of fellow hibakusha.

He, like other survivors, required a certain amount of psychic numbing in order to carry out his mission, or even to function in general. Catastrophe requires one to call forth what Freud referred to as a "protective shield." This one city official was struggling to sustain an equilibrium between numbing and feeling.

His overall response followed much of the classic myth of the hero who experiences a "call to greatness," undergoes a "road of trials," and brings to his people special knowledge he has acquired, in this case of death and a path to rebirth.

Another impressive emergent leader was a professor of ethics who was also seriously injured by the bomb and lost the function of one eye. Having been closely associated with the Japanese military regime, he spoke of "atoning for my mistakes" by working for peace. He embarked on various forms of humanitarian help for other hibakusha and for world peace. But he eventually decided to simply sit before the Cenotaph (the monument to the victims of the bomb) in the Hiroshima Peace Memorial Park whenever any nation tested nuclear weapons, encouraging others to sit by him.

While the number of those who joined his vigil was limited, he felt that "there is something special about sitting in Hiroshima in front of this Cenotaph . . . on behalf of the dead, 200,000 people [and their] 'voiceless voices.'" When a little girl asked him, "Can you stop it by sitting?," he proclaimed publicly that "a chain reaction of spiritual atoms must defeat the chain reaction of material atoms." That was the more visionary meaning he gave for his action, while fully understanding the challenge of the girl's question. He became prominent in Hiroshima as a man of moral integrity who represented a version of hibakusha commitment to combatting the weaponry.

During a return to Hiroshima in 1975, I heard that he was sitting by the Cenotaph in response to someone's nuclear testing somewhere, and I went there and sat down beside him. I wanted to make clear that I shared his concerns, admired his actions, and wished to join him in antinuclear protest.*

These initial emergent leaders were struggling to move hibakusha beyond debilitating victim consciousness. And over the years a number of hibakusha began to speak out as people with a special knowledge of atomic catastrophe. They spoke in Hiroshima, throughout Japan, and in various parts of the world, and could claim survivor wisdom about the nuclear threat to humankind.

In 1956, hibakusha joined together to form an umbrella

---

* I had previously made clear my commitment to peace but had refrained from any form of activism in order to have access to people in Hiroshima whose attitudes differed from mine. But I had essentially completed my research project and felt comfortable engaging in this modest act.

group called Nihon Hidankyo (Japanese Confederation of A- and H-Bomb Sufferers Organization) whose organizing statement described a sequence from victims to death-driven survivor-activists.

That organizing statement included demands for a hibakusha aid law, while containing a mantra of "No more hibakusha!" and "No more Hiroshimas, no more Nagasakis!" The Hidankyo group would later take its own extensive survey of the extended hibakusha community, emphasizing continuing anxieties and the experience of discrimination in marriage and work.

Overall, Hidankyo demanded that the people of the world "never . . . take your eyes off Hiroshima and Nagasaki; listen to what hibakusha are saying; know the realities of the damage caused by atomic bombs." They condemned the suppression of information concerning the full impact of the atomic bomb by both Japanese government authorities and the American Occupation. In the Hidankyo statement, hibakusha do not deny their sense of victimization and death anxiety, but declare them to be a valuable source of energy for the group's antinuclear crusade.

The statement expresses a survivor mission, explicitly on behalf of the dead: "Our resolve is nothing but that of the silenced voices . . . of the people who died a miserable death at the moment of the bombing, of those who died of horrible A-bomb disease." The message is that these survivors recognize their debt to the dead and are not only acknowledging that debt but acting on behalf of its payment.

That survivor mission marks a transformation for hibakusha from passivity to activism: "Up until now we have kept our silence, hid our faces, scattered ourselves, and led [the] lives that were left to us, but now . . . we are rising up. . . . We have acquired the courage to stand up." What results is "a sensation of 'resurrection'" and then the power of survival: "We are glad that we are alive."*

A very significant emergent leader was to appear long after my Hiroshima study. Setsuko Thurlow experienced the atomic bomb at the age of thirteen when working as a member of the student mobilization program at army headquarters, 1.8 kilometers from the hypocenter. She lost eight members of her family, experienced symptoms of acute radiation, and for months was terrified of developing

---

* It must also be said that a great deal of the energy toward reconstituting Hiroshima came from outsiders arriving from different places in Asia that had been occupied by Japan.

the dreaded and often fatal purple spots of invisible contamination.

Her activism began in 1954 with her response to the extensive damage and radiation effects caused by the American testing of hydrogen bombs in the Marshall Islands. She later participated in Peace Boat, an organization that provided ships on which hibakusha could travel the world to disseminate their antinuclear message.

She became an organizing member of the nuclear umbrella group ICAN (International Campaign to Abolish Nuclear Weapons), which was awarded a Nobel Prize in 2017 for its achievement of a United Nations treaty that rendered illegal not just the use but the creation and stockpiling of nuclear weapons. The treaty of course referred to hydrogen bombs, which could have as much as a thousand times the destructive power of the two atomic bombs used in 1945.

Thurlow gave one of the Nobel reception speeches, in which she called forth details of her own survival as a metaphor: "I hear a man saying, 'Don't give up! Keep pushing. . . . See the light? Crawl towards it.'" She has received recognition and awards for her survivor activism and call to renewal: "This is our passion and commitment for our one precious world to survive."

Through such survivor activism, both Hiroshima and Nagasaki have become iconic cities recognized throughout the world as geographic and psychological centers for disseminating nuclear truths. Hiroshima has had greater visibility, but Nagasaki has produced its own powerful words, including those expressed in a memorial ceremony: "The bomb fell first on Hiroshima, then on Nagasaki. Let Nagasaki be the *last* place it falls."

3

The Struggle for Meaning

Chaim Kaplan, in a diary he kept from the Warsaw Jewish ghetto, wrote, "The worst part of this ugly death is that you don't know the reason for it. . . . The lack of reason for these murders especially troubles inhabitants of the ghetto. . . . We feel compelled to find some kind of system to explain these murders." He observed prisoners to feel that "if there is a system, every murder must have a cause; if there is a cause nothing will happen to me since I myself am absolutely guiltless." He went on, "People do not want to die without cause."

Survivors can only emerge from immobilizing "victim consciousness" by finding some form of meaning and significance that can help them grasp what they have endured.

The beginning of the quest for meaning, the key to the survivor experience, is the *imprint of death*. The survivor experiences a jarring awareness of the fact of death and can be confronted, in particularly disturbing ways, with his or her own mortality. Any prior illusion of invulnerability, individual or collective, has been shattered.*

---

* There are exceptions in which survivors, having lived through a deadly force, can speak of themselves as newly invulnerable, but such examples are rare, and even when they occur, the assertion tends to be brittle and subject to self-doubt.

That death imprint affects all future behavior. It occurs whatever one's preexisting psychological traits. It can vary in intensity according to the force of the catastrophe, and people bring different degrees of vulnerability to it. But it is a signature event of catastrophe, inseparable from the death anxiety that haunts the survivor experience.

For some catastrophes with especially massive killing and dying, such as occurred in Hiroshima and Auschwitz, there are no prior experiences or images to call upon for meaning. What in one's life would enable one to envisage a single weapon destroying an entire city, or a camp whose function is systematic murder and working to death those allowed at least temporarily to survive? That is why Hiroshima and Auschwitz survivors can talk about their ordeal as a profound learning experience, emphasizing the value of that experience for them.

At the same time, they require dramatic forms of psychic closing off, or what I came to call psychic numbing, in order to deal with both the immediate cruelty and the prospect of their own deaths. Psychic numbing resembles other psychoanalytic defense mechanisms such as repression, isolation, derealization, and denial, but it is unique in being concerned exclusively with feeling and nonfeeling.

In that way survivors are quickly initiated into a struggle over what and how much to feel.

Survivors, as victims of extreme trauma, can also undergo a form of what I call *doubling*, the creation of a seemingly separate traumatized self, necessary for adaptation (for instance, a numbed self), while still holding on to elements of one's prior, less immobilized, pre-traumatized self.

Both "selves" are of course part of one's overall self but can be functionally almost independent. That is why former Auschwitz inmates, when asked how they managed to survive, could say, "I was a different person in Auschwitz." Or "I simply stopped feeling."

Some, in surviving, can be near heroic in their achievements while remaining extremely vulnerable. One need only look at the example of Primo Levi, the extraordinary writer who was an Auschwitz survivor and provided as nuanced a description of what occurred in that camp as any we have, but who retained sufficient inner despair to take his own life years later in connection with the fatal illness of his aged mother.

A central post-traumatic task of survivors is to reconstitute the self: the two halves in connection with doubling, and the separate pieces that have broken off and require reintegration. The process is part of an overall struggle to derive knowledge from trauma.

The survivor's early quest for meaning is bound up with a sense of debt to the dead. Some find that debt unpayable and remain fixed in a sense of guilt for having "abandoned" the dead and themselves remained alive. But others can call forth what I have called an *animating relation to guilt*, a propensity to transform it into the *anxiety of responsibility*.

They then can bear witness to the catastrophe on behalf of the dead and take on a survivor mission to combat the lethal force.

In this way survivors can embark on a project to extract meaning from absurdity, vitality from massive death. They can work toward an overall formulation of the disaster— what it consisted of, how it came about, and what its significance may be. Such a formulation helps orient the self to the new reality, toward taking in what really happened. Hibakusha did that in forming groups that made known the details of their catastrophe, even as they involved themselves in the reconstruction of Hiroshima.

I also worked with a very different group of survivors, antiwar American veterans of Vietnam. In their opposition they found *meaning in the meaninglessness* of their war.

That meaning, in turn, could convert them into what I came to call "antiwar warriors," whether in carrying out their own often fierce and highly influential protest movement, or in intense participation in peace movements initiated by others.

But survivors can also give vent to angry despair and even wish that their dreadful fate be shared by the rest of humanity. For instance, in Elie Wiesel's *Night*, his searing memoir of his time in Auschwitz and Buchenwald, he describes a transient wish "to burn the whole world." Similarly, in Hiroshima, I was told of the kind of underground wish among a number of hibakusha "that atomic bombs fall all over the world." Or that, noting the new arms race, they fall on American and Russian cities.

In an equally despairing mode, a hibakusha who had been remarkably active in helping many to survive experienced a transient wish for Hiroshima's total destruction by catastrophe. Strikingly, Shinzo Hamai, the heroic city official who, more than anyone else, has been associated with Hiroshima's eventual recovery, experienced such a moment of despair when Hiroshima underwent extensive flooding six weeks after the bomb: "The city looked like a huge lake. . . . I felt as though this was the final burial! Suppose the flood waters were never to recede, and Hiroshima were to remain drowned forever? In that case, I thought, so much the better. I said this to myself in all seriousness."

In this case, an extraordinary leader hit rock bottom, not just with total helplessness but with a momentary wish that the catastrophe would be so decisive that he would be relieved of his pain and the endless sense of futility in struggling against it.

But what he saw and felt also clarified his awareness of the depth of the Hiroshima disaster, a clarification he could draw upon to sustain his own efforts at keeping people—including himself—alive. That kind of emergence from despair has considerable relevance for us now.

Americans, and others throughout the world, continue to struggle over meanings given to Covid-19. At this writing, the pandemic has killed more than 6.5 million people, including more than 1 million Americans. The virus stalks everyone at various levels of consciousness, even as it evolves and changes. It is nowhere and everywhere, and its omnipresence can be experienced as a supernatural entity. We find it difficult to bring reason to such an invisible but deadly force, especially one that has delayed symptoms and sometimes no apparent symptoms at all.

This aspect of Covid-19 response has some psychological resemblance to Hiroshima survivors' fear of invisible contamination from radiation effects. In both cases the strangeness and unpredictability of the experience renders death unnatural, indecent, and absurd. Though in Hiroshima, those symptoms were mostly confined to one city and its surroundings. Not so with Covid-19. Also the coronavirus is physically contagious, and radiation effects are not.

Covid-19 is especially confusing because each of us can be both in danger and dangerous to others. Each of us must constantly struggle with not only a death imprint but with our own deadliness. While vaccines have diminished much of that deadliness, it has by no means been entirely eliminated.

A closer historical model for Covid was the Black Death, or "Great Dying," of the bubonic plague, which swept through Europe and Asia during the fourteenth century. Accounts of the Black Death include monstrous alteration of bodily substance and a contagion that led people to experience the plague as close to all-enveloping. They led to such statements as "The sailors, as if accompanied by evil spirits, as soon as they approached the land, were death to those with whom they mingled." And "The contagion was so great that one sick person, so to speak, would 'infect the whole world.'" That is, "A touch, even a breath, was sufficient to transmit the malady." These are images of death, carriers who can also take on a quality of supernatural evil.

For an even closer model we might look to the 1918 influenza pandemic, which killed at least 50 million people worldwide, including an estimated 675,000 people in the United States, making it the deadliest pandemic in modern history. The H1N1 virus, known at the time as the "Spanish flu,"* was global in reach, was largely spread through respiratory droplets, and was combatted with similar pre-vaccine prevention tactics such as the use of face masks, hand washing, social distancing, and quarantining.

Meaning depends upon memory. The failure to sustain active cultural memory of the 1918 flu pandemic, to hold its details in our collective imagination, raises important questions about legacy and learning from the past. That

---

* There is no universal consensus about where the 1918 influenza strain originated. Spain became associated with the virus because it was neutral in World War I; it had no need to suppress information on cases in the manner of warring countries, who feared seeming weak if illness and deaths were high.

failure to retain such crucial historical knowledge left us psychologically vulnerable to Covid-19, which we perceived as totally unpredicted and random, having no relationship to anything before it.

I have already distinguished between severely affected Covid survivors, haunted by direct or family experience of the illness, and everyone else, whose more muted death anxiety can belie our own status as survivors of what constantly threatens us.

An obstacle to finding Covid meaning is the widespread anxiety caused by physical and psychological exhaustion in doctors, nurses, and medical assistants. Contributing also to that anxiety have been deficiencies in personal protective equipment and the availability of medical facilities in general, and the simultaneous fear and uncertainty about opening schools and businesses providing vital services. That anxiety has also been sustained by varying attitudes toward the vaccine, including considerable resistance to it.

There are ebbs and flows in our awareness of Covid danger and the degree of collective anxiety about it. But variants like Delta and Omicron, the subvariants that emerge from them, and fear of additional contagious and potentially deadly variants in the future give the pandemic a feeling of endlessness. That constant instability and uncertainty conflict with a deep collective yearning to return to "normal."

Patients in psychotherapy provide a valuable window to changing patterns of Covid anxiety. Prior to the vaccine, patients' voices could become suffused with dread when they mentioned the virus. They felt stalked by it and unable to find the inner resources to deal with its ubiquitous effects. Some were strongly upset. For instance, one patient was described as dreaming nightly of forgetting to wear his mask, or of the band on his mask breaking, or of being out of hand sanitizer. Another, an elderly cancer survivor, was so terrified by the fear of contagion that he refused to enter the elevator of his building.

But with the availability of the vaccine, the anxieties of patients have changed. Patients tell how their expectation that the vaccine would resolve the issue has not been realized, and about their frustration in connection with the general confusion that prevails about what is safe and what is not, about which precautions are still necessary under what conditions.

Therapists themselves cannot be immune to these fears and frustrations, whether having to do with their own and family members' exposure to variations of the virus, or to uncertainties about it they share with patients.

Unmanageable death anxiety can lead to a general *apocalyptic aura*—an all-consuming narrative of the end of the world. Here Covid-19 joins with what I call the apocalyptic twins of nuclear and climate threat.

Nuclear fear can be caused by the weapons themselves, by threats of their use, by meltdown in energy reactors, or by residual radiation effects in sites where the weapons were made or tested. Such nuclear fear has become a model for other large threats that endanger the human future. The omnipresent Covid-19 threat readily connects with the *imagery of extinction* we associate with nuclear weapons.

Indeed, such ultimate threats tend to merge in the individual mind as an overall sense of world ending. In a study I conducted with Charles Strozier in the early 1990s, entitled "Nuclear Fear and the American Self," we found climate and nuclear anxieties to be closely interwoven. Psychological associations between them could occur within the same thought, sentence, or phrase. Covid-19 has entered that same apocalyptic realm, connecting with existing world-ending threats.

In the basic Judaic and Christian apocalyptic narrative, the total destruction gives rise to a newly purified world. But that apocalyptic narrative can be variable. With any of these three ultimate threats—Covid, nuclear, and climate—the apocalyptic promise of world purification becomes hazy, so that there may be very little hope for what follows the world-ending catastrophe. Apocalyptic auras attract gurus and disciples who may attempt to find hope in the end of the world itself, as they seek to be, as the American philosopher William James put it, "melted into unity." That is, to blend into one another in their apocalypticism.

Also part of the apocalyptic aura has been the disturbing imagery of climate disaster: unprecedented drought and fires, and hurricanes and tornados that have filled our screens, along with ever more grave scientific warnings. Such environmental destruction has always been inseparable from nuclear apocalypticism.

Moreover, many embrace biblical references that become associated with a prophecy of apocalypse: "fire and brimstone" suggests nuclear explosion, while the great flood that brought about Noah's ark is a parable of something resembling climate change. In the book of Genesis, God declares that "I will cause it to rain on the earth for forty days and forty nights." The book of Revelation describes hailstones and droughts and darkness and lethal earthquakes in which "the sun became black as sackcloth, the full moon became like blood" and "every mountain and island was removed from its place" and "the rivers . . . became blood."

The Covid-19 pandemic also has biblical connotations in the ten plagues of Egypt created by God in order to convince the Pharaoh to allow the Israelites to depart from slavery, including turning water to blood, boils, locusts, and death of the Egyptian firstborn.

Other social anxieties that might seem remote from Covid amplify the apocalyptic aura: the struggle for racial justice that includes the Black Lives Matter movement; the uncontrollable American "gunism" resulting in mass shootings, particularly of schoolchildren; the increasingly extreme attacks on abortion and reproductive rights; the anti-LGBTQ sentiment and legislation; the experience of inflation and fear of recession; the embrace by rightists of violence and threats of violence; and the overall assault on democracy and its pivotal principle of free elections.

Our minds may not separate out these threats so much as experience them as an all-pervasive threat to existence.

Covid anxieties both contribute to and are enhanced by the prevailing apocalyptic aura.

These apocalypticized fears can be associated with a feeling of loss of control of our lives, loss of closeness to others, loss of our grounding. We sense that we are being forced to change but we cannot quite grasp what that entails. Recognizing what is happening to us in these catastrophes becomes itself a project and even an act of courage.

As terrible events become commonplace, we experience a version of what I call *malignant normality*. We can recognize—and to some extent accept—the existence of extreme threats as part of our world, and carve out our individual routines. Indrajit Samarajiva, a writer who lived through the end of the Sri Lankan civil war, speaks of "the numbing litany of bad news, the ever-rising outrages. People suffering, dying, and protesting all around you, while you think about dinner . . . it's Saturday and you're thinking about food while the world is on fire. This is normal. This is life during collapse." And "that's the thing about regime collapses: Even while the government is falling, people still get married and have kids and go to bars and watch TV."

As we obtain partial control of the virus via vaccination

and other measures, death anxiety may diminish at least enough to enable us to explore imaginative narratives other than the apocalyptic one.

Covid-19 survivors are doing just that, insisting on making themselves heard as a people suffering from the effects of a concrete ailment. But we face a deeply troubling impediment, which has to do with widespread rejection of the truths of catastrophe.

4

Rejecting Catastrophe
and Survival

No one I met in Hiroshima denied that a catastrophe had occurred. That all too painful recognition enabled them, over time, to look toward a contrasting moral universe in which life is valued or at least tolerated and actions have consequences. No wonder that survivors of catastrophe are sometimes called "collectors of justice."

But what happens when a major segment of society *refuses to acknowledge the basic truths of a catastrophe*, as is the case in America today with the Covid-19 pandemic?

For societies to cope with catastrophe they must first recognize its existence. To reject a catastrophe is to reject the survivor state and to bring about profound social confusion that can give rise to violent conflict.

Since the beginning of the Covid pandemic, Trump and the radical right embraced a political stance of downplaying it as a catastrophe. This has contributed to the extraordinary number of American Covid deaths. Dr. Deborah Birx, the former Trump administration's coronavirus response coordinator, has estimated that more than 130,000 American lives could have been saved during the early stages of the pandemic if the Trump administration had followed epidemiological principles and implemented proper mitigation measures.

Trump did support a fast track for scientists working on a vaccine, convinced as he was that it would enhance his chances for reelection.* But later, after the vaccine was provided, he refrained from mentioning the word "vaccine" because by then it had become anathema to people in his political base.

As president, Trump's response to the pandemic was largely characterized by what I call his *solipsistic reality*, based on what his own self seeks and needs, however removed from accepted standards of evidence. More than that, he sought to impose that solipsistic reality on American society in general.

For example, on January 22, 2020, Trump wishfully declared, "We have it totally under control. It's one person coming in from China, it's going to be just fine." And on February 10, as it was becoming clearer that the virus was not under control, his comment was, "It looks like by April, you know, in theory, when it gets a little warmer, it miraculously goes away." He said this in spite of the pan-

---

* Trump signed off on the intense vaccine initiative, called Operation Warp Speed, seeking to deliver a vaccine before the November 3, 2020, presidential election.

demic's increasing deadliness, substituting negation of the danger for desperately needed forms of mitigation.

Combined with that rejection of pandemic truths was Trump's early scapegoating (and racist) claim in his reference to the "China virus." Since then he and the radical right have come to a more general accusation that methods imposed to contain the pandemic are part of a liberal plot to restrict individual freedom. In stark contrast to hibakusha, whose truth telling about their catastrophe contributed to recovery, Trumpist negation of Covid-19 truths has consistently and dangerously stood in the way of individual and social healing.

In this rejection of the reality of the pandemic they have been joined by many anti-vaxxers—people with a resistance to vaccines in general or to the Covid-19 vaccine in particular—and by white supremacists and paranoid conspiracists such as QAnon believers.

There has been overlap and mutual stimulation among all these groups. What emerges is a *subculture of righteous conspiracism* that minimizes the pandemic and rejects the very effective vaccines that have been developed. Some righteous conspiracists go so far as to compare mandatory masks with the Nazi requirement that Jews sew the Star of

David onto their clothing, an equation that may unconsciously refer to the death anxiety associated with both.

There have of course been many contradictions in this pandemic rejection. There have been cases in which people, seeking to retain their Trumpist/right-wing political identity, have received the vaccine but have done so secretly or even in disguise, while others who were sickened by the virus have gone to their deaths rejecting its reality. Trump himself has expressed these contradictions, as when he suggested that his followers should take the vaccine while also declaring that "I believe in your freedoms 100 percent"—meaning, of course, the freedom, even encouragement, not to take it.

There are various shades of gray in Covid-19 anti-vaxxers. They include people who have had no objection to childhood vaccinations but, influenced by a drumbeat of disinformation, have come to view Covid vaccinations as a violation of their personal bodily integrity.

Some prominent athletes, who in this case bring intense focus to their bodies as the source of their remarkable achievements, have confused the vaccine with a claim of their right to bodily control. What is not part of their moral equation is the risk of endangering others, particularly their teammates, and also themselves. But that ethically fraudulent claim of bodily integrity can have a certain appeal nonetheless.

This rejection of the reality of the pandemic and of basic methods of preventing transmission of the virus is an example of one of the many situations in which a claim of American individualism becomes a source of extreme danger to other Americans. Here many leaders, especially religious leaders, have been remiss in failing to assert principles of concern and love for one's neighbor, and for communal well-being. In the United States these principles would be mainly Christian, but they are espoused by all major religions.

Without such articulation, more people in the society are likely to turn to aggressiveness and violence as means of suppressing their death anxiety.

No one can completely *deny* the existence of Covid-19. It has killed more than 1 million Americans and is visibly physical and biological in its illnesses and deaths. But those righteous conspiracists can and do *reject* the pandemic or its full measure.

In that rejection they move toward a cultlike, self-enclosed community, even if geographically dispersed, insisting on its claim to the ownership of reality. One of the ways in which Covid-19 rejectors defend their falsehoods is to confuse and challenge others' recognition of the omnipresence and lethal threat of the pandemic.

Yet since Trumpists and other conspiracists experience the catastrophe they reject, they too need to find some form of meaning. They not only resort to scapegoating but *create imagined catastrophes of their own*. They embrace right-wing antigovernment paranoia and conspiracy theories such as "the genocide of white people" and the "great replacement" of white Americans by non-white minorities.

At the center of such imaginary catastrophe is the fierce embrace of the Lost Cause mythology surrounding the American Civil War. That mythology emerged from the struggle among survivors over the collective meaning given to any war. According to the noted Civil War scholar David Blight, the Lost Cause interpretation of the American Civil War attempts to "cast . . . the Confederate defeat in the best possible light . . . [and] . . . nostalgically celebrates an antebellum South of supposedly benevolent slave owners and contentedly enslaved people, and downplays or altogether ignores slavery as the cause of war."

The losers "needed explanations and stories in which to

embed their woe, their loss, and their hatred." Within this distorted mythology, the Ku Klux Klan could be seen as a defender of a noble cause and the leading Southern general Robert E. Lee was accorded with "near sainthood" and celebrated as "the country's truest Christian soldier."

That Lost Cause behavior has included a mass carving in the stone mountains of Georgia of a bas-relief of three Confederate generals, with words such as "sacrifice and valor" and somehow a quote from the American revolutionary hero Patrick Henry.* Lost Cause behavior was intensified during the Obama administration and reflected, in the words of philosopher Susan Neiman, "the fury that had been rising since a black family moved into the White House."

Since the Civil War, Lost Cause celebrations in Southern towns have been framed in religious terms, and "Lost Cause theologians conceived the south as a nineteenth century Jesus, innocent and martyred but destined to rise again."

---

* Patrick Henry actually played a leading role in creating the Bill of Rights. He opposed slavery as a "lamentable evil" and confessed to his contradiction as a slaveholder: "I will not, I cannot justify, [owning slaves]." Henry was sometimes called the "father of the founding fathers."

Lost Cause mythology is an alternative catastrophe. It contributes to the creation of a counterfeit universe in which a significant segment of our current society believes, which includes the Big Lie about the stolen election and the rejection of the truth of the Covid-19 pandemic.

In this way Trumpists can view themselves as martyrs to their versions of truth. Within their false claim of reality, they can see themselves as *survivors after all*. They can embark on an *equally false survivor mission* to "stop the steal" and reinstall Trump as president, which was precisely the mission of the insurrectionists who attacked the Capitol on January 6, 2021.

The Big Lie about the election becomes (to use a neurological term) the final common pathway for those self-designated survivors. They are on a psychological treadmill in which extreme measures, often violent, can become necessary for sustaining their perverse survivor meaning and mission.

The radical right frequently invokes its martyrs, militia members killed while combatting government forces. The falsehoods and distortions concerning those martyrs could join the conspiracist (in writer-activist Todd Gitlin's words)

"Vortex [of] the Birthers, Whitewater, 'Travel Gate,' and Vince Foster conspiracy theorists, 'Death Panel' enthusiasts, 'lock her up!' chanters, scientist hunters, and other flat earth factions."

One source of this violent, conspiracist behavior is death anxiety. Death anxiety is among the most painful of human experiences, and much of the psychological work in our society is now connected with avoiding it. Death anxiety is primal and inhabits one's entire being. Violence, an ever-ready means of fending off death anxiety, is more external and considerably less painful (though perhaps never fully successful).

Imagined catastrophes and false survivor missions can eclipse the actual catastrophe of the pandemic. Yet Trumpists and other Covid-19 rejectors are threatened by the virus like everyone else, even if their politics and their subculture require them to deny its danger. They must therefore call forth considerable psychic numbing in order to suppress their own death anxiety. Masks and vaccine injections become fraught because they are reminders of the deadliness of the virus.

When insurrectionists invaded the Capitol on January 6,

2021, and physically attacked Capitol police, they were seeking to reverse the outcome of the election but may also have been struggling to contain death anxiety.

The Trumpist-cultist assault on reality is fueled by what the political theorist Nancy Rosenblum and I have called a *perversive immoralism*: various forms of indecency, viciousness, and recklessness about consequences. That immoralism is most lethal in connection with Covid-19. Indeed, throughout the pandemic, Trumpists have colluded with the virus—have held rallies and meetings that inevitably became sources of Covid outbreaks while rejecting and actively resisting behavior (masks, distancing) that could mitigate such outbreaks.

Trumpists, along with other rightists and cultists, go further in what can be called "riding the virus." By that term I mean exploiting it, often attacking messengers of truth, and deriving political capital from their version of it. Riding the virus involves different forms of falsification. We now know that Trump himself had contracted the virus much earlier than he had publicly acknowledged, had exposed people to it at a super-spreader event at the White House, and also exposed Biden and others to it during the final presidential debate. We know as well that when Trump was later hospitalized due to Covid-19, he had been much closer to death than revealed publicly. This was an extreme, aggressive, even homicidal way of riding the virus.

That immoralism was also evident when Trumpists were in power and sought to "heal" society and return it to full functioning by means of exposing Americans to illness and death. The weak could be sacrificed; there could be a mystical "herd immunity"; the robust would be fine. By offering up those at highest risk from the virus, Trumpists rendered them expendable.

There are certain parallels between Trumpist behavior and Nazi policies that are worth noting. The Nazis also sought to "heal" their society by killing. And much of early Nazi energy came from a false survivor mission. They could deny the actual catastrophe of defeat in the First World War by means of stab-in-the-back mythology: the claim that the German army did not itself lose World War I but was sabotaged, mostly by Jews as well as by Communists, socialists, and other "traitors."

Nazi mythology included a "cult of the fallen" that rendered slain German soldiers a sacred community of martyrs to the German cause. Nazis claimed to join in that sacred community, to the extent that chairs could be left empty at meetings, and the names of the fallen called out.

The Nazi cult of the fallen had specific parallels to the Lost Cause of the American South and the martyrdom of dead Confederate leaders and soldiers. Though the Nazis were generally anti-Christian, they could nonetheless connect the presence of the "fallen" with the "passion and resurrection of Christ."

In their perversion of meaning, the Nazis created an origin story of redeeming the dead and joining them. Within this false witness, Hitler became their version of a survivor-redeemer, invoking his own combat experience in World War I. He claimed that while suffering from the effects of poison gas he had a vision of becoming a great leader who would restore the German nation. And he dedicated *Mein Kampf* to the *Blutzeuge*, or "blood witness," of the subsequent martyrs who were killed in 1923 in the failed insurrection known as the Beer Hall Putsch. This "blood witness" was converted into survivor rage directed at the Treaty of Versailles for placing the blame on Germany for World War I while rendering the nation impotent by stripping it of military power.

More generally, false witness is at the heart of much

victimization. It creates what I call *designated victims*: the Jews in Europe, African Americans in this country. Where there is extensive trauma, the scapegoating imagery of survivors can be in the service of relieving death anxiety. The dominant group exploits its designated victims in carrying through its own psychological work.

When Trumpists sought to "heal" American society by opening it up completely despite the raging pandemic, they rendered other Americans—notably the elderly and immunocompromised—their designated victims.

Victimization can also take the form of accusations of post-catastrophe criminality, generally made against longstanding designated victims in a society. What is alleged to have occurred *after* the catastrophe becomes inseparable from blame for the catastrophe itself. Such accusations can be prominent among survivors of any disaster.

For instance, immediately after the Great Kantō Earthquake of 1923, which leveled the city of Tokyo, ethnic Koreans were rounded up and killed in what became known as the Kantō Massacre. Vigilantes were often helped by police and other authorities in both the killing and the "speaking tests" uncovering the accents of ethnic Koreans, but often mistakenly killing Chinese and Japanese from outer regions whose accents were considered suspicious. Koreans were accused not so much of causing the earthquake but of taking advantage of the disaster to commit arson, robbery, sabotage, rebellion, and the poisoning of wells.

That image of the poisoning of wells was also an accusation made against Jews during the plagues of the Middle Ages. The image is a way of finding meaning not only by the scapegoating of others but also by viewing those being scapegoated as reversing the life-giving aspect of water and rendering the water deadly.

With the appearance of social media, the old pattern of post-catastrophe victimization takes on a new dimension. Now anyone who wishes to have a voice has access to technology that takes "the most incendiary, most hateful messages and put[s] them in front of the biggest possible audience." Through these media channels, Trumpist immoralism can be wildly exacerbated.

The investigation of the Facebook Papers, which uncovered internal documents from 2019 to 2020, helped bring the scope of this exacerbation to public attention. The investigation revealed that "anti-vaccine commentators" dominated Facebook pages, along with drug cartels and human traffickers. This was consistent with Facebook's availability to QAnon conspiracy theories, election falsehoods, false cancer cures, and Holocaust denial. Facebook's remedial steps have had limited effect.

In August 2020, while Covid cases were surging throughout the country, a report revealed that the top ten producers of "health misinformation" had managed four times as many views on Facebook as had the top ten sources of authoritative information.

President Biden was in no way exaggerating when he declared that the Facebook falsehoods were "killing people." He could have added that they were also contributing to the Big Lie about the election, and to the January 6 insurrection.

The social media problem is part of what can be called our *attention society*. Michael Goldhaber, who uses the term "attention economy," asserts that "attention . . . not information is the natural economy of cyberspace." And when you have attention "you have power."

He declares that "Trump has been a near perfect product of an attention economy [or attention society]," and that the January 6 Capitol insurrection resulted from "thousands of influencers and news outlets that, in an attempt to gain fortune and fame and attention, trotted out increasingly dangerous conspiracy theories on platforms optimized to amplify outrage."

Goldhaber is telling us that Trumpist lethal expressions of false meaning and mission are rendered profoundly dangerous by the attention they receive in an attention society.

And yet that same attention society can also give expression to what Václav Havel, the remarkable Czech writer and revolutionary, called "living in truth." For Havel, that was the remedy to any systems of "living a lie." Havel helped create an expanding community of people who managed to live as if free, whatever the malignant normality they confronted. That is what he meant by "the power of the powerless."

Such truth-telling communities have their own vulnerabilities. But in America they still constitute a majority, whatever the prominence of the disruptive minority of pandemic and vaccine rejectors. A dramatic example of such a truth-telling community is the Select Committee to Investigate the January 6th Attack on the United States Capitol. In both its content and its attention to factual truth, that committee has combatted Trumpist solipsistic falsehoods. It does so by (in Nancy Rosenblum's term) *enacting democracy*.

We are still living through the Covid-19 catastrophe. The full range of true expressions of survivor meaning and mission is by no means entirely clear. Meaning and mission remain uncertain because of the elusive nature of the threat, the diversity of attitudes and responses. Especially harmful—and deadly—are the ideological extremes of the radical right, which drive them to reject and even violently oppose the best methods of prevention and treatment.

For some survivors, however, there has been a powerful emergence of meaning and mission. I have in mind the groups that put forward their own experience with the disease in their demand for greater societal awareness, particularly of the effects of long Covid.

The politicization of the pandemic has had deadly consequences that we must still reckon with. We are all involved in a death-haunted struggle against false witness, and on behalf of living in truth.

5

The Mourning Paradox

One cannot function as a survivor without undergoing mourning. But mourning can itself be problematic, often resisted, and sometimes associated with violence. The process of mourning is at the heart of our struggle to consolidate survivor meaning and embark on a survivor mission of renewal.

Survivors mourn for people they have lost, and also for lost homes, streets, and possessions. They mourn for their lost former selves, for their innocence toward death. The mourning process is a struggle with grief, with the experience of pain and anguish of loss. Mourning also includes efforts at repair, at reconstituting a damaged psyche. That sequence of loss, anguish, and repair is constant in human experience.

That process can be both urgent and protracted because it is so important for coping with death anxiety. Without it, death anxiety can dominate one's life and become an obstacle to renewal.

Survivors' grief is bound up with an insistent quest for meaning. What was it that brought about the loss? And how can that knowledge help one overcome that loss?

Descriptions of mourning are mostly individual, and the phenomenon has held important sway in psychoanalytic thinking from Freud to the present. But in the case of larger catastrophe, mourning can be widely shared in response to collective loss. Such collective mourning does more than bring together many individual experiences. It can enable a society to harness its social and political currents in the service of post-catastrophe recovery.

Mourners, however, can be immobilized by their struggle. As the humanist Kathleen Woodward has put it, "By asserting we have lost someone, do we not also mean that we *feel lost* ourselves, that in our grief we have lost our sense of direction?"

Generally speaking, there is no moving beyond loss without some experience of mourning. But what if mourning is somehow impaired or disrupted? To be unable to mourn is to be unable to enter into the cycle of death and rebirth so central to all mythologies and religious narratives. It is to be unable to "live again."

Psychoanalysts Alexander and Margarete Mitscherlich raise important questions about the significance of mourning in connection with collective catastrophe in Hitler's Germany. The Mitscherlichs considered postwar Germany a nation of survivors unable to come to terms with the love they had experienced for their Führer. Most Germans prefer to forget how intense those feelings were, how infused with imagery of shared virtue and of national purification and revitalization.

The Mitscherlichs were asking what it means to discover evil in what one has lost—and, by implication, in oneself. How does one reconcile that evil with the sense of nobility one had originally associated with one's love? Is it then possible to mourn? If so, for whom and for what? What is the relationship of guilt and responsibility to mourning, or not mourning? What are the collective consequences of the inability to mourn?

The Mitscherlichs regularly observed in their postwar German psychoanalytic patients "the defense against collective responsibility and guilt—guilt whether of action or of toleration." They emphasized that virtually all segments of German society, notably people in industry and the professions, "had given the regime their definite and enthusiastic support; but with its failure they regarded themselves as automatically absolved from personal responsibility." It is precisely this "intensive defense against guilt, shame, and anxiety" that rendered them unable to mourn the loss of the Führer. One cannot mourn a loss one does not acknowledge. The Mitscherlichs associated that denial of responsibility and inability to mourn with national German stagnation in the political and social spheres.

But there are many situations other than the one the Mitscherlichs describe that express the potential consequences of the inability to mourn. There is a well-known case history in existential psychiatry entitled "The Attempted Murder of a Prostitute," in which a previously inconspicuous young man shoots a prostitute. Contributing to his violence were complications of mourning for the recent death of his father, as well as the early childhood loss of his mother. The author, Roland Kuhn, quotes a phrase from the lyric poet Rainer Maria Rilke: "Killing is one of the forms of our wandering mourning." Even without killing, struggles over mourning can be associated with anger or rage.

Jacques Lacan, the often brilliant (and at times a bit mad) French psychoanalyst, wrote about Hamlet as an example of one who was not so much unable to mourn as unwilling to mourn because he neither wanted to end his confrontation with his father's death nor take action in connection with it. In that way Hamlet preferred to remain psychologically "stuck."

There is also a refusal, rather than an inability, to mourn

in the Trumpist and radical right's reaction to Covid-19. The political need to reject the catastrophe precludes mourning for its losses. That refusal to mourn is a refusal to change or to recognize change in others. What can result is unrelieved pain on a large scale and diminished social capacity to cope with the virus.

There can be dead ends to the mourning process in which a belligerent defensiveness can give way to violence. Such mourning-related violence can also be an expression of revenge, as in the case of some jihadist groups. The general principle is that of angry mourning associated with violence.

An example here is the largest recorded atrocity of the Vietnam War. Although not usually viewed this way, the My Lai massacre of March 16, 1968, was an act of angry and violent mourning. Within a few hours nearly five hundred Vietnamese civilians—women, old men, children—were slaughtered by soldiers of Charlie Company of the Americal Division. Two days before the massacre a funeral ceremony had been held for a sergeant named George Cox, who had been blown to pieces by a "booby trap"—a fake artillery shell he had been trying to dismantle.

There had been increasing deaths and injuries caused by

such devices, and by hit-and-run attacks by an often invisible enemy. But Cox's death was particularly devastating. He was an older man with extensive combat experience and had been something of a father or older-brother figure many in the unit had depended upon for support and guidance.

There was a chaplain present at the funeral ceremony, and the eulogy for Cox was given by the company commander, Captain Ernest Medina. The eulogy brought his listeners close to tears, and then went on to become a military pep talk. Medina was quoted as saying, "Now we're gonna get our revenge. Everything goes." And "there are no innocent civilians in this area." The men also sensed that he "wanted a big body count" to present to his own superiors, who had pressured him at an earlier meeting to "get more aggressive." In this way, murderous military policies combined with angry collective mourning to create an atrocity-producing situation. With such a combination, even men who are quite ordinary and not particularly prone to brutality or violence are capable of extreme atrocities.

During the massacre, the soldiers kneeled and crouched while shooting, "like some kind of a firefight with somebody." In this shared illusion of combat, their gunning down of old men, women, and babies enabled them to feel that they had finally engaged an elusive enemy and gotten him to stand up and fight.

For some the killing seemed to bring psychological relief, though only temporarily: "I lost buddies . . . so after I done it [the massacre] I felt good. But later on that day it kept getting to me." And there was something of a feeling that "the killing even made some kind of sense," and "seemed like the natural thing to do"—also that after it the company "became more effective." The mourning process had gone awry. This confused violence in connection with mourning was an expression of larger struggles with the meaninglessness and absurdity of the war.

In my earlier writing about My Lai I spoke of the Vietnam War's "moral inversion" and "absurd evil," suggesting that the mourning experience was inseparable from this moral issue. More recently this view has been given further structure in psychological discussions of "moral injury" and "moral repair."

Antiwar Vietnam veterans I interviewed came to express their emergence from the counterfeit moral universe of Vietnam with active opposition to their own war. That required different, nonviolent forms of mourning, associated with their country's military mission in Vietnam.

On April 23, 1971, Vietnam veterans engaged in a particularly poignant and angry expression of such nonviolent mourning when they stood at the foot of the Capitol building and threw their medals back to the country (including its military and political leaders) that had awarded them. Someone played taps and each veteran then gave his name, rank, and military awards, as he tossed the medal as one would a baseball, football, or hand grenade.

Descriptions of the event mentioned "raw fury and deep sadness" but also considerable catharsis in the action. The veterans shouted such things as "This is for my brothers!" or "This is for Private Jim Smith, killed at Da Nang, for no goddamn reason!" An antiwar group of Gold Star Mothers joined them in throwing away awards received by their dead sons.

I could observe veterans' struggles with mourning during the "rap groups" we shared. These included critical explorations of the belligerent machismo that had contributed to their unquestioning version of patriotism. One could say that they mourned for their former view of their country's virtue, its claim to always seek peace and fight only to defend itself and to do so fairly. Confronting that loss was crucial to the impressive degree of individual change that many could achieve. These antiwar veterans were struggling with what Freud called "the work of mourning," which always includes a debt to the dead. Significantly, their mourning was shared as they responded to, and evoked memories in, their fellow mourners.

Mourners' involvement with the dead can rarely be simple or straightforward. Their simultaneous debt to, and separation from, the dead is a key to survivor behavior. Survivors can make clear, as hibakusha did, that their debt to the dead is a source not only of credibility but also of constructive energy. At the same time, we have also seen that hibakusha have felt the need to separate themselves from the dead in order to assert their own life power.

In Hiroshima, mourning was complicated by Japanese cultural beliefs that related the "debt" to unsuccessful attempts to prevent the dying. In Japanese tradition a body was thought to become a corpse at the moment its soul—its life principle—separated from it. One way of preventing or delaying the soul from departing, or to call it back when it had just left, was to offer water to the person nearing death. That cultural belief was painfully involved when hibakusha sought to keep dying people alive by offering them water.

According to these same cultural beliefs, once the soul was thought to have departed, the dead body became something close to a phobic object, defiled and defiling. Sometimes the dying person could be kept in isolation during the final hours, "so that the foulness of death would not affect other members of the community." The rice bowls that had been used by the dead person could even be destroyed for the same reason.

In most cultures there is some version of a dread of corpses, which must be quickly buried or otherwise disposed of. In the case of those who die through violence, or prematurely, there is a danger that they will become "homeless souls" who represent a threat to the living. The suggestion here is that these "improper" deaths cannot be adequately mourned, and that they therefore cannot become "immortal souls" that replenish the flow of life.

In large catastrophes where there is an absence of corpses, and of individual graves, mourning can be profoundly difficult. That was very much the situation in Auschwitz and Hiroshima. In both cases there were attempts to record the deaths of individual people, but those efforts were over-whelmed by the dimensions of the catastrophe.

With the Covid-19 pandemic, mourning has been ren-dered more difficult by the isolation of medical facilities and the inability of family members or close friends to be present with the sick and the dying. Also contributing to the difficulty is the extensive psychic numbing that may take the form of dismissing the pandemic, refusing to wear masks, and participating in large gatherings. Indeed, vari-ous forms of psychic numbing are found in all the catastro-phes I have been discussing.

In Auschwitz and other camps, the most extreme psy-chic numbing—the most extreme evidence of the inabil-ity to mourn—was the so-called *muselmänner*, so named because Muslims were thought by the prisoners to make a total surrender to the environment. The *muselmänner* had lost their capacity to mourn, or to feel anything at all. They became, as Primo Levi put it, "An anonymous mass, continually renewed . . . of nonmen who march and labor in silence, the divine spark dead within them, already too empty to really suffer. One hesitates to call them living: one hesitates to call their death death. . . . If I could enclose all the evil in our time in one image, I would choose this image which is familiar to me: an emaciated man, with head dropped and shoulders curved on whose face and in whose eyes not a trace of thought is to be seen."

The *muselmänner*, as the ultimate expression of numbed inability to mourn, could experience none of the anger that recent observers have found to be present in mourning. Intense forms of psychic numbing could thus negate the life process in general.

The Covid-19 catastrophe has created its own widespread need for mourning. As early as May 2020, the historian Micki McElya, an authority on the "politics of mourning," stressed that yearning in an article entitled "Almost 90,000 Dead and No Hint of National Mourning." She wrote that although then-president Trump repeatedly returned to the idea that America was "at war" with the virus, there was "a conspicuous absence of any collective mourning at all [for coronavirus 'war' causalities]." Moreover, she added, "shared grief brings people together like little else." She went on to quote Judith Butler's observation that "we have to consider the obituary as an act of nation-building."

McElya stresses, as I do, that the mourning must be collective: "This is not to minimize the personal trauma . . .

but we do need to acknowledge the collective toll we all share in this grief—including those of us who have not experienced an immediate loss. A nation of 'warriors' honors its fallen."

Collective mourning is more complex and more difficult to identify than its individual expression. But it is crucial to recovery from any catastrophe. To understand it, we need to consider the larger context of social and political currents. Those currents have to do with widely shared attitudes about what has happened to one's group or community. Collective mourning involves steps toward reconstituting the life of a community that has undergone loss.

The collectivity we call the nation, led by its president, should be primarily concerned with people's living and dying. But Trump, as president, only said, "I don't take responsibility at all."

I find it natural to look at these larger dimensions because I have been doing that throughout my psychohistorical work. I have made use of the experience of individuals as an approach to collective tendencies. But I have also required a focus on collective behavior and thought as necessary for understanding the meaning of what people say about individual experience.

Collective mourning always combines the psychological and the political, making use of older religious and cultural currents. To be sure, those broader influences are present in individual mourning, and in that sense all mourning is importantly shared. But in collective mourning the sharing is the essence of the process.

One of the best examples of collective mourning has been provided by an extraordinary monument, known to most simply as "the Wall." The Vietnam Veterans Memorial is a V-shaped structure of polished black granite—actually two walls—four hundred feet long, sunk into the landscape next to the Lincoln Memorial and containing the names of Americans killed or missing in Vietnam: originally 57,939 names and ultimately 58,320 after additions made in 2018.

It is a very quiet memorial, stark and heartbreaking. In its tabulation of death and pain and nothing else, it manages to eliminate political and military considerations. Vietnam veterans go there to acknowledge the death of specific comrades, in many cases "rubbing" their names on paper with wax crayons or graphite pencils—as is frequently done when making a pilgrimage to graveyards.

When the Wall was officially dedicated on Veterans Day,

November 11, 1982, there was a combination of joyous celebration and healing ritual. During a four-day period, there was a vigil at the National Cathedral at which all the names were read. There were floats and bands and joyous forms of nonmilitary marching, in some cases while pushing wheelchairs of injured comrades.

Naming the dead, *all* the American dead, has profound psychological importance. It immediately connects each individual death with the larger catastrophe of collective loss.[*]

A number of people have pointed out that there is something wrong about the absence of Vietnamese names on the Wall, as an estimated million Vietnamese people died in that war. The Wall, then, is limited to American-centered mourning, but the kind of mourning that allows for psychological openings on behalf of the losses of the former enemy.

There is an accompanying Vietnam Women's Memorial near the original. There have also been many replicas of the

---

[*] I was moved to find that I have a personal connection, however indirect, to the Wall project. I have been told by a veteran associated with the project that they were influenced by my work on Vietnam.

Wall in various cities, including a smaller "Traveling Wall," which, in the spirit of the original, has an educational function. And there is a separate statue of three soldiers meant to look heroic, created to satisfy those made uneasy by the Wall because they feared, with some justification, that it would contribute to antiwar feelings.

The Wall was clearly created as a public structure, made possible by an act of Congress, but it provides private space for each individual mourner. That private space, rather than being lost in the collectivity, contributes to an entire nation's struggle to recover from catastrophe.

The psychological and the political are always intertwined. That interaction can be toxic, as in the case of Trump, or it can lead to a constructive dynamic in which minds are eased in ways that enable more people to accept the truth of actual catastrophe. Building such a life-affirming "virtuous circle" was the intent of one of the first acts of Biden's presidency.

On the eve of Biden's inauguration, he and Vice President Kamala Harris led the country in a national moment of collective mourning: a dramatic vigil in which four hundred lights surrounded the Lincoln Memorial Reflecting Pool to honor the four hundred thousand American lives that had then been lost to Covid-19. Americans across the country were encouraged to join in the memorial by lighting candles in their windows and ringing bells—and to light up city buildings, including the Empire State Building in New York City, as expressions of participation in the event.

Biden and Harris conducted a second ceremony the following month to memorialize crossing the threshold of five hundred thousand deaths, in which the president mentioned "survivor's remorse." He and Jill Biden, and Harris and Doug Emhoff emerged from the White House at sundown and stood at the foot of the South Portico as a Marine Corps band played "Amazing Grace." Biden spoke emotionally, again emphasizing his theme: "To heal, we must remember." He added, in reference to his own personal losses: "I know all too well . . . that black hole in your chest. You feel like you're being sucked into it. The survivor's remorse. The anger. The questions of faith in your soul."

There have been other important forms of collective mourning. Religious rituals for mourning are still very much with us, even if in many groups their practice has diminished. Secular forms of mourning are often improvised but can retain elements of religious tradition. There has also been an outpouring of artistic renderings of mourning. An example has been the work of Suzanne Brennan Firstenberg, who created an installation of thousands of flags planted in the National Mall, each to represent a coronavirus death.

Firstenberg's piece was reminiscent of the AIDS Memorial Quilt, conceived in 1985 by the gay activist Cleve Jones. First consisting of panels that each contained the name of an AIDS victim, it eventually became a gigantic fabric quilt that has been displayed on the National Mall and throughout America and the world. Jones spoke of how the Quilt "could . . . reveal the humanity behind the statistics."* In 2020, a special virtual exhibition of the Quilt was disseminated throughout the country to help people face the pain and loss from the Covid-19 pandemic.

There have also been musical events for Covid-19 in many different places, emphasizing Samuel Barber's "Adagio for Strings," which begins with a single B-flat and has

---

* The HIV/AIDS epidemic has killed more than 35 million people since its beginning in 1981, making its mortality second only to that of the 1918 flu epidemic in recent history, and considerably greater than the Covid pandemic to date.

often been played for funerals, including those of Albert Einstein, John F. Kennedy, and Franklin D. Roosevelt.

Covid memorials have been created online that collect and share "public content created by people who were exposed to Covid deaths, with personal messages of love."

And there is talk about a national Covid memorial, where that might be placed, how it would look. The leading architect Daniel Libeskind speaks of "an urgency because there are people here now. Their memory is a fire burning in their hearts"—rejecting a national policy of waiting for twenty-five years after a historic event for a memorial to be built.

One activist survivor organization, Marked by Covid, has been campaigning for physical monuments and a federally recognized national Covid-19 memorial day. Its founder, Kristin Urquiza, insists that "we owe it to the million people who lost their lives to remember and pass down to future generations the hard truth of our lived experience to prevent a tragedy like this from ever happening again." She says, "We cannot forget this tragedy."

Insofar as we can collectively mourn, these deaths are acknowledged to belong to all of us.

6

Activist Witnessing

How does a society emerge from catastrophe and find paths to renewal? Covid-19 responses, despite many difficulties, suggest their own version of an answer. That answer has to do with witnessing as part of the ethics of survival.

I have mentioned groups of severely affected Covid survivors, including those whose relatives have suffered or died from it. They have organized to become what has been called by the *New York Times* "a vast grass-roots lobbying force that is bumping up against the divisive politics that helped turn the pandemic into a national tragedy." Those groups include Marked by Covid, Covid Survivors for Change, Young Widows and Widowers of Covid-19, and Survivor Corps. Such groups actively hold meetings, speak out, and write declarations and articles in which they demand recognition of their suffering—calling for others to say: "We see you, we hear you, we stand with you, and we care."

As with earlier movements involving disease or bodily attack—such as AIDS survivors and survivors of Hiroshima—these immediate Covid-19 survivors began with a focus on their own needs but quickly turned to questions of meaning and demand for action. One survivor group has called for a special commission to investigate the pandemic in order to help prevent its recurrence. And we have seen how another has proposed the establishment of a permanent Covid memorial day.

An organization with the striking name Body Politic started a Covid-19 support group after its founder and a board member fell ill with the virus. The group engages in advocacy campaigns for Covid-19 patients and long-haul Covid. It stresses "intersections of wellness and social justice." Another group, called Long Covid SOS, has written a notable letter to the prime minister, health secretary, and others involved in health policy in the UK calling for recognition of "the needs of those with Long Covid."

Still another group, the Patient-Led Research Collaborative, describes itself as a "self-organized group of long Covid patients working on patient-led research around the Covid experience." Those patients are themselves "researchers in relevant fields—participatory design, neuroscience, public policy, data collection and analysis, human-centered design, health activism—in addition to having intimate knowledge of Covid-19." The group has produced studies on long Covid, one of which is called "What Does Covid-19 Really Look Like?" and another, "Characterizing

Long Covid in an International Cohort: Seven Months of Symptoms and Their Impact."

A healthcare network called Kindred has emerged with an app that utilizes new technologies to enable survivors to connect more readily with Covid research in general. Their goal is "provide opportunities for anyone interested in contributing to research to do so," because "collectively our experiences can inform research, and advance healthcare in ways that are urgently needed." Since the government is unable to track down the details of all of these cases, such groups provide a supplement that helps overcome the limitations of ordinary public health methods.

All these groups and others involve immediate Covid survivors who insist on bringing their special knowledge to bear on the larger society. The impact of such knowledge is far from certain, as is the response of American society. But since the majority of Americans have been infected with Covid-19, there is every likelihood that these survivor groups will rapidly expand. And there is the hopeful possibility that this expression of survivor wisdom will also resonate with the more distant Covid survivors who make up the rest of our society.

These Covid-related groups constitute a survivor-based

movement in which bearing witness to truths about the virus becomes a basis for activism.

The groups expose the malignant normality of continuously understating Covid danger and the failure of American society to recognize the full scope of the pandemic. In doing that they are rejecting false narratives claimed to be social truths. As patients become more professional and professionals become patients, distinctions between them blur and witnessing becomes more clear. Professionalized patients sometimes find themselves in conflict with established epidemiologists, but even then the ensuing conversation can be a source of further knowledge and witness.

Survivors, scientists, and survivor-scientists can all become versions of what I call *witnessing professionals*. As such, they make use of their experience and knowledge to reveal the profound dangers of the virus. They come to resemble research scientists who expose and combat global warming, and also physicists who expose the danger of nuclear weapons and oppose their stockpiling.

My own experience in Hiroshima also applies here. When I carried out that research I was intent on conducting it scientifically, making use of a protocol in my interview method. I also tried to maintain the ethical standards of my profession by obtaining consent and remaining sensitive to the psychological state of the people I interviewed, while avoiding any approach that might be harmful to them.

Yet I came to recognize that there was a larger ethical dimension that had to with making known to the world what these survivors told me. I was learning what the bomb did to individual people and to an entire city. I did not yet have words for that dimension, but it entailed taking in as much as possible of the atomic bomb experience described to me and retelling it from a psychological and historical perspective.

I would later understand this as bearing witness to what I, as a professional, encountered in that city. The survivors themselves were the immediate witnesses; I was a witness to the witnesses. In the process I came to realize that the more disciplined I was in my interviews, and in my presentation of their content, the more effective my witness would be.

Of course that Hiroshima story was focused on nuclear threat. But climate change has also been a catastrophic threat that has called forth significant professional witness. And we are experiencing such witness with Covid as well.

Early on I began to suspect that nuclear and climate threats were closely related. I recently discovered an article, "Hiroshima and the Ultimate Pollution," among my papers deposited at the New York Public Library. Written in the late 1960s, I had never published it but had used it in talks I gave. The article emphasized our new capacity to destroy our natural world. I referred to the "breakdown of ecological balance" and suggested that we use such terms as "poison," "deterioration," "degeneration," and "starvation." At that time, I had no grasp of the work on climate change scientists were only beginning to carry out. What I did recognize was that nuclear weapons posed a profound threat to the larger human habitat. That combined fear of nuclear catastrophe and the destruction of the human habitat had also been expressed in the terrifying early rumors of Hiroshima being unable to sustain life of any kind.

To be sure, Hiroshima is the most extreme kind of destructive event; it immediately lends itself to various forms of witness. But we have learned that the effects of climate change can have their own extremity. Climate scientists have identified some of those effects as very much present in our immediate world and as posing a threat to human civilization over the course of this century.

Surely, the situation requires of us an ethic that confronts this threat to the human species and most other species as well. That broader ethic enables us to confront truths having to do with the destruction of the human habitat and extend previous commitments to ways of preventing or mitigating that looming catastrophe.

The sequence of American response to nuclear threat can also teach us much about the role of witnessing professionals. Malignant nuclear normality has been present since the bombs appeared in the world: in their actual use as weapons in Hiroshima and Nagasaki; in narratives (especially by scientist-strategists Herman Kahn and Edward Teller) of fighting and winning nuclear wars;* in the duck-and-cover drills for schoolchildren (ducking under desks and covering their heads with pieces of paper) to avoid nuclear injury; in a Harvard-sponsored book, *Living with Nuclear Weapons*, that included the willingness to use the weapons under certain conditions; in the dubious rescue technology of using antiballistic missiles to intercept nuclear weapons

---

* Kahn described how an American president might say to advisers, "How can I go to war—almost all American cities will be destroyed?" and receiving the answer, "That's not entirely fatal, we've built some spares."

(the Strategic Defense Initiative, or Star Wars), though it actually encouraged first-strike mentality; and in the "modernization," often miniaturization, of the weapons to make them more usable.

For sustaining nuclear normality, psychiatrists and social scientists were enlisted for a government program in 1956 to help Americans diminish their fears of the "threat of annihilation" and to enable them instead "to support national policies which might involve the risk of nuclear warfare."

But from the beginning there also emerged witnessing professionals who exposed and contested malignant nuclear normality. The first group of these consisted of scientists involved in producing the bomb, who sought to prevent its use on a human population. One of them, the biophysicist Eugene Rabinowitch, told of walking the streets of Chicago in the summer of 1945 and "imagining the sky suddenly lit up by a giant fireball . . . skyscrapers bending into grotesque shapes . . . until a great cloud of dust rose and settled onto the crumbling city."

Rabinowitch was calling forth an anticipatory image, taking on a survivor function in advance of a catastrophe. He joined others in preparing an urgent written plea that the bomb be used only in demonstrations and not on human targets. They were not able to stop the atomic bombing of Hiroshima and Nagasaki, but they provided the origins of the scientists' movement that, after the war, devoted itself to bearing witness to profound nuclear dangers.

The physicians' antinuclear movement, in which I have participated, considers itself a successor to that of the scientists.[*] As medical professionals, we have had a very simple message: This time we can't patch you up or help you recover. We're doctors, we would like to do that, but hospitals will be destroyed, there will be no medical facilities or equipment, and in any case you will probably be dead and so will we.

Our national group, Physicians for Social Responsibility (PSR), had public meetings in major American cities. Our international group, International Physicians for the Prevention of Nuclear War (IPPNW), did so in cities throughout the world. American and Soviet physicians were at the heart of the movement, and at each meeting

---

[*] There have of course been other groups, such as the Committee for a Sane Nuclear Policy, which reached much greater numbers of people and prepared American and international groups for what we as physicians have to say.

there was a seriously humorous toast offered by one of them from either country: "I drink to you and the good health of your people and your leaders—because if you survive we survive, if you die we die."

That planetary ethic was at the heart of the physicians' movement and was conveyed by Eugene Chazov, the leader of the Soviet delegation, to his friend Mikhail Gorbachev, then premier of the Soviet Union, who quickly embraced it. Chazov had teamed up with his fellow cardiologist Bernard Lown, the leader of the American delegation, who initiated the international movement. Lown had no such friend in power; our movement was anathema to the Reagan administration.

This principle of mutual security—of human security— has been at the center of all antinuclear movements but had special impact when put forward with the professional authority of physicians throughout the world. It was the basis for the Nobel Peace Prize awarded in 1985 to IPPNW.

Vladimir Putin directly rejected that planetary ethic when he threated to use nuclear weapons in connection with his invasion of Ukraine in 2022. While such threats had been made by others in the past, including the United

States, there had been no equivalent sense of nuclear danger since the Cuban Missile Crisis of 1962, after which a planetary taboo had prevailed.* Putin's rejection of that taboo shocked a world that had come to depend upon that broader ethic. Here the authority of hibakusha could be asserted in a public statement by Hidankyo condemning the Russian invasion of Ukraine and Putin's "attitude of willingness to use nuclear weapons and even to fight a nuclear war."

The climate change movement calls forth that same planetary ethic. This has particular relevance for us during the Covid-19 pandemic because it too remains active and there is lethal interaction between climate and Covid in their effects on vulnerable people.

Because we are earthlings, we are born into climate change and its version of malignant normality. We then face an ultimate absurdity: by merely continuing with our current energy practices, particularly our use of fossil fuels, we will ultimately destroy our civilization. We needn't start

---

* There have been various nuclear threats made by North Korea, India, and Pakistan, but these were not considered as immediately dangerous as the risk posed by either the Cuban Missile Crisis or Putin's behavior during the Ukraine war.

a war or make use of any level of weapons. We needn't do anything other than what we are already doing to endanger the future of our own species, and much of our civilizational destruction will take place within this century. This ultimate absurdity creates the most all-encompassing expression of malignant normality that we face.

The witnessing professionals who emerge from among climate scientists include physicists, chemists, geologists, and a variety of atmospheric scientists. Their witnessing task has been documenting and demonstrating the profound and diverse climate dangers of global warming.

Climate scientists differ from their nuclear counterparts in having done nothing as a group to create the problem. But they have done everything to identify the danger. They were at first quite alone in their witness, emerging from their various scientific professions to create the very concept of a climate scientist. A watershed moment in American consciousness was physicist James Hansen's 1988 testimony before a Senate subcommittee on global warming.*

---

* Unfortunately, Hansen has since come out strongly, and more intellectually loosely, for a large-scale nuclear energy solution, which suggests that valuable professional witness can be followed up by less disciplined and potentially harmful advocacies.

The bad news is that the dedicated efforts of committed climate scientists have not succeeded in sufficiently influencing political leaders to take the steps necessary to effectively combat climate change. The good news, however, is that over recent decades there has occurred what I have called a "climate swerve," a shift in the mindset of the American population from denial and rejection to a recognition of the actual causes of climate change and the need for mitigating action.

The international event that epitomized this climate swerve was the United Nations Climate Change Conference in Paris in November and December 2015. Whatever its failings, that conference was an expression of species unanimity. Rather than legally bound commitments, its greatest achievement may well have been its collective state of mind, its near universal witness to the threatened state we share as members of a single species.

From the time of that meeting, those supporting malignant climate normality have been on the defensive, so much so that then President Trump experienced fierce national and international responses to his efforts to extricate the United States from that agreement. Those efforts were met with outrage throughout this country, including that of mayors and governors, and with equally strong pro-test from leaders and officials throughout Europe.

Malignant climate normality has its own instability. No longer is it possible for anyone to avoid knowing in some part of his or her mind that the climate threat exists. Many suppress and resist these truths because they contradict their worldview, their identity, their party politics, their own vested interests, and their donors' and supporters' demands. It is more a matter of climate *rejection* than denial. That rejection is still widely embraced by right-wing groups but at times has been a political liability. Climate scientists, though frustrated by resistance to change, have nonetheless had considerable psychological and political impact.

With Covid-19 too, the task of witnessing professionals has been crucial and ongoing and has had its own complications. I have mentioned the professionalization of knowledgeable Covid survivors. Among witnessing professionals are the physicians and medical personnel who follow the lead of epidemiologists in providing hands-on treatment to Covid-infected people. And that hands-on treatment can involve dangerous exposure to the disease and related anxiety and exhaustion. When these caregivers are referred to as heroes, we understand it to mean that they are protecting the larger society at considerable personal cost. Importantly, their own excruciating witness can be enhanced by the organized groups of survivors that are emerging.

The public face of the Covid-related witnessing professionals has been Anthony Fauci, who spent decades as the director of the National Institute of Allergy and Infectious Diseases. As a prominent American epidemiologist, he mentored five administrations of presidents and the general public with his insistent narrative of scientific truth—most recently of Covid-19, including close attention to our changing understandings of the virus and its spread.

As chief medical adviser to the president with the Biden administration, Fauci was tireless and constant in telling us where we stand with the virus and what we could and should do to overcome it. He has also been courageous in coping with vicious conspiratorial attacks in which this most consistent opponent of the virus is accused of having secretly created it. In truth, Fauci has probably made as great a personal impact on American society as has any scientist in recent history.

Yet even with his extraordinary contributions to our society, Fauci encountered a particular problem that bears more discussion. While he was serving on the Trump administration Covid team, Trump could partly silence him by forbidding him to appear on various media, notably on prominent television programs. In that way Trump and his followers could sustain their deadly confusions in connection with the virus, and in some degree make use of Fauci as a respectable cover for their behavior. This would not have mattered so much if it had not occurred during a period of staggering American deaths resulting from Trump's mishandling of the Covid virus.

Fauci and other government scientists were caught in a classic dilemma of how long one should stay connected to wrongheaded and dangerous leadership in order to have influence from within, as opposed to separating oneself from that dangerous leadership in order to oppose it freely. At least one prominent epidemiologist, Irwin Redlener of Columbia University, recognized this conflict and urged that Fauci and other government scientists "step down [and] speak out about the pressures that have been put on you by Donald Trump [and] stand up for public health, science, and for saving lives by refusing to work for presi-

dent Donald J. Trump." But Fauci rejected the suggestion because he equated resigning with "quitting," with
"walk[ing] away."

Witnessing professionals, like all others, cannot avoid
moral and political questions in relation to who they serve
and how much genuine witness they are able to offer.

That dilemma can be better understood by looking at
the historical emergence of the idea of witnessing professionals in general. As early as the twelfth century, there
emerged the idea of "professing" one's religious convic-
tions, one's vows as a member of a religious order. But over
subsequent centuries, as society became more secularized
and more technicized, professional guilds and societies
were formed that were devoted to perpetuating craft and
technique rather than religious faith. So much so that this
technical emphasis came to be associated with ethical neu-
trality. Modern professionals could become hired guns,
serving the highest bidder.

The development of what we call professional ethics
has imbued our work with standards of decency but has
in no way addressed present threats to human civilization.
Our ethical task now is to extend that decency to our species, which we can only do by committing ourselves—as

witnessing professionals and simply witnessing citizens—to preserving it, and preserving other species as well. In that way our species becomes our sponsor, and witnessing activists can emerge from all levels of society.

We still retain our more immediate and local identities—whether as Christians or Muslims, as Italian, Jewish, or African Americans, as Russians or Nigerians. But those immediate identities take on a connection to the human species as a whole. We may move in and out of that planetary identity, but the continuous world-destroying threats do not allow us to forget it.

The ethic required, whether for Covid, nuclear, or climate threat, is one of "professing" and acting upon our commitment to humanity. Active witness is not so much the creation of a new entity as the embrace of an ethic necessary for our era.

7

The Legacy of Survivors

With all catastrophes, survivors' expression of direct witness is limited by the length of each of their lives. But even after their deaths, that witness can provide a powerful legacy for future generations.

Dictionaries define a legacy as "a tangible or intangible thing handed down by a predecessor; a long-lasting effect of an event or process" and "something handed down from an ancestor or predecessor or from the past." An example given as early as 1579 was "Our Sauiour Christ . . . left bequeathed vnto vs the Legacie of eternall lyfe."

But how does a legacy take shape? What can it achieve? And are there dangers of losing it?

Ortega y Gasset, the early-twentieth-century Spanish philosopher, spoke of "the concept of the generation [as] the most important one in the whole of history," which provides history with an "internal lack of equilibrium" so that it "moves, changes, wheels, and flows." That generational flow can in some degree be derailed by the distortions and falsehoods of social media that affect everyone. But subsequent generations can nonetheless embrace original survivor knowledge to confront catastrophic threats of their own era. The significance for us of Ortega y Gasset's concept is that of ever-new engagement and transformation of the original survivor message.

For instance, the story of a city's destruction put forward by hibakusha can reverberate in Japan and elsewhere in the world for subsequent generations threatened not only by nuclear weapons but also by other catastrophes such as climate change and Covid-19.

But how are experiences of catastrophe transmitted after immediate survivors are gone? They can be passed down, directly and informally, through word of mouth in families and communities, and sometimes taught limitedly in schools. But they can also be given more public structure in memorials and commemorative events, as well as in artistic and literary expressions of the survivor as creator.

Such a legacy can become geographically rooted, as in the case of Hiroshima's designation by the Japanese parliament in 1949 as a City of Peace. The designation followed strong advocacy by Shinzo Hamai, Hiroshima's first popularly elected mayor and himself a hibakusha. It could even be accepted by the American Occupation authorities, despite their general suppression of discussion of the bomb and its special features.[*]

What resulted was the Peace Park close to the bomb's hypocenter, which came to contain the Cenotaph, the official monument to the victims of the bomb, along with a Peace Memorial Hall, a Peace Memorial Museum, a Children's Peace Monument, and a Peace Bridge and Peace Road. Hiroshima University, not too far away, was rebuilt and envisioned as an intellectual center for peace.

But subsequent developments revealed some of the difficulties in creating a legacy. Questions were raised by Japanese officials about how much to include in the museum about Japan's militaristic past and its attack on Pearl Harbor.[†] Those questions reflected the varying interpretations of the ambiguous inscription on the Cenotaph: "Rest in Peace. The mistake shall not be repeated." (What was the "mistake," was it only a "mistake," and who made the "mistake"?)

---

[*] Some believe that the Occupation did so in order to diminish the criticism it was receiving for censoring discussion of the atomic bomb.

[†] Although the great majority of the people killed by the bomb were civilians, Hiroshima had contained a military base.

Those conflicts were also expressed in relation to the Atomic Bomb Dome (or Peace Dome), which consists of the remains of one of the few reinforced concrete buildings in Hiroshima and became a receptacle for ambivalence. Some hibakusha I interviewed emphasized its importance. One spoke of it as "a kind of warning, the only thing that remains [to suggest] that such a thing once happened." Another declared that, "without it, we would tend to forget the event completely . . . [it represents] a responsibility coming from my being alive."

Others disagreed and emphasized its relationship to pain for hibakusha themselves. One spoke of "a sense of dread, and that building [a dome] . . . seemed dark, gloomy, and horrible"; advocating that "it would be better to tear the dome down right away, rather than increase this grief." I heard one particularly imaginative suggestion that "we should figure out the exact hypocenter . . . and leave it devoid of anything at all . . . in order to symbolize nothingness [because] . . . such a weapon has the power to make everything into nothing."

Some advocated for a decision by nondecision: neither tear the dome down nor permit it to stand indefinitely but instead wait until it begins to crumble on its own and then simply remove it. That changed when, in 1965, construction began on a nine-story office building right next to the dome, which rendered it almost invisible, causing renewed efforts by Hiroshima officials and others to undertake reinforcement of the dome for the purpose of "eternal preservation." The survivors who emerged from victimization could point to the dome as suggesting, quietly and powerfully, the destruction of the city around it.*

Hamai went on to establish a traditional ceremony to commemorate the bomb experience, to recall it to our collective memory and at the same time celebrate survival and renewal.

Some hibakusha could be critical of this highly public, ceremonial event, in keeping with a frequent survivor distrust of versions of commemoration or artistic re-creation that stray from the literal details of the catastrophe, viewing such efforts as "an insult to the dead." But the August 6 statement from the international City of Peace, expressed

---

* Since 1996, the Dome has been a UNESCO World Heritage Site, protected by Japanese law.

in a speech by the mayor, could annually disseminate to the world a message of the experience of unprecedented destruction followed by a plea for peace.

Commemorations of catastrophe are necessary. They are an act of remembrance that can pass along to others some of the truths of that catastrophe. They require a recapitulation of the trauma, which can be painful to survivors and their families, who may be still grieving. To commemorate is to share memories, however painful, and can contribute to collective renewal, with survivors in the vanguard.

The AIDS Memorial Quilt (as part of the National AIDS Memorial) has evolved into one of the most enduring commemorations, now the largest community folk art project in the world, with nearly 110,000 names sewn into its fifty thousand cloth panels. The Quilt has been made virtual and is viewed regularly throughout the world. Similar online Covid-19 remembrances take on resemblances to this project and to other officially designated national memorials such as the Vietnam Veterans Memorial, the National September 11 Memorial & Museum, the Pearl Harbor National Memorial, and the National Lynching Memorial (officially the National Memorial for Peace and Justice).

A stunning new technology has recently emerged for preserving the direct witness of survivors for future generations. Dimensions in Testimony utilizes a method in which a survivor is closely interviewed and painstakingly recorded so that a powerful and highly realistic image of that survivor can be programmed to answer just about any question that can be asked—whether about the details of their ordeal or any other aspects of the survivor's life. The virtual survivor brings unlimited energy to answers provided and can continue to do so after that actual survivor has died and for potentially infinite future generations. The conversation can cause the questioner to experience what Freud referred to as the "uncanny," having to do with the breakdown of the distinction between life and death, and that sense of the uncanny may contribute to rendering the experience unforgettable.

Who can forget the voice of Pinchas Gutter, a Holocaust survivor, whose testimony was given in 2014 at the age of eighty-two, telling the questioner, "Now that you have heard my story . . . you're actually part of me because I've handed over part of me to you. . . . I would like you, number one, to remember it. . . . I'd like you to treasure it . . . to use it as a vehicle to teach others to make the world a better place . . . to not do what I went through . . . that is my greatest wish."*

The project is part of the University of Southern California Shoah Foundation (created in 1994 by the prominent film producer and director Steven Spielberg) and has been successfully pursued in various Holocaust museums. The technology is far from perfect—there can be problems in connections with questions and answers—but it does bring powerful enhancement to the legacy of immediate survivors for future generations.

But whatever the brilliance of Dimensions in Testimony, it cannot replace the need for new generations to develop and carry through their own version of engagement, whether with Holocaust survivors or survivors of catastrophe in general. That legacy will importantly contain physical monuments and various forms of commemoration.

The absence of legacy and commemoration can have a considerable cost. Consider once more the worldwide

---

* At the time of this writing Gutter himself was still very much alive at ninety, but it was his virtual image that received and responded to questions.

influenza pandemic of 1918 with its 50 million deaths, and subsequent disappearance from cultural memory. A British social scientist, Martin Bayly, who studied UK records concerning that pandemic, "couldn't find any evidence of any public commemoration whatsoever." According to Bayly, "the absence of commemoration meant that it did fade away in public memory, in the writing of history."

Crucial to survivor legacy is the creative retelling of catastrophe through literature and the arts. As the postwar German novelist Heinrich Böll put it, "The artist carries death within him, like the good priest his breviary."

That was strikingly the case with the French writer Albert Camus. In his Nobel Prize acceptance speech of 1957, Camus drew upon his experience in the French Resistance in the Second World War when he asked the question, "Do you know that over a period of twenty-five years, between 1922 and 1947, seventy million Europeans—men, women, and children—have been uprooted, deported, killed?" The "do you know" meant: Do we let ourselves remember? Do we permit ourselves to feel?

That question could be repeated to include Ukrainians and Russians in 2022, and also Asians, Africans, and other non-Europeans over recent decades. Camus viewed such things, in the words of one of his biographers, "as a scandal that he himself finds impossible to evade." He was telling us that we live in a landscape of holocaust, in which literature must emerge and life must be lived. On that basis (and without in any way equating ordinary life to the experience of holocaust), we all have in us something of the witness of the survivor.

In both his personal life and his work, Camus was sensitive to the survivor's potential for confronting a death immersion and seeking from it a measure of insight. He emphasized a particularly painful individual survival of the death of his close friend René Leynaud: "In 30 years of life no death reverberated in me like this one." And in his play *Caligula*, Camus put forward the most dangerous kind of individual survivor response to catastrophe: a protagonist who, after the death of his sister, must kill and continue to kill in order to sustain his own unending life, his immortality.

In his great novel *The Plague*, Camus's central character is a physician who, in the face of death and suffering, does nothing heroic but simply lives out his calling to provide medical and spiritual help. As this physician-narrator explains, "What had to be done and would assuredly have to be done again in the never-ending fight against terror and its relentless onslaughts by all who are unable to be saints but refusing to bow down to pestilence, strive their utmost to be healers."

Our contemporary pandemic makes clear that such a commitment to healing can indeed become heroic, because, as we have noted, doctors and other medical personnel must put themselves at risk from Covid-19 in order to carry out their healing function and protect the larger society.

Camus and other creative survivors have often sought their survivor illumination while working in theater groups, drawing upon the community that theater provides to explore their innovative confrontation with death. A towering example here is that of Samuel Beckett, who, like Camus, also did dangerous work in the French Resistance. In his writings, Beckett managed to render death-dominated, rock-bottom experience a source of life-enhancing energy. His depiction of despair became a form of artistic breakthrough that nurtured human culture throughout the late twentieth century.

Another striking example of survivor imagination is Kurt

Vonnegut's novel *Slaughterhouse-Five.* The book devotes only a few beginning pages to Vonnegut's exposure, as a prisoner of the Germans, to the British and American fire-bombing of Dresden. And most of those pages are about his inability to write "my famous Dresden book" for a period of twenty years. Yet he states that the book:

> is so short and jumbled and jangled . . . because there is nothing intelligent to say about a massacre. Everybody is supposed to be dead, to never say anything or want anything ever again. Everything is supposed to be very quiet after a massacre, and it always is, except for the birds.
>
> And what do the birds say? All there is to say about a massacre, things like "*Poo-tee-weet?*"

He makes clear that all that follows in the book is the consequence of his death immersion and survival in Dresden. Vonnegut himself remained alive by finding shelter in a meatpacking room within a larger slaughterhouse and then, over a six-month period, was assigned the task of collecting and burying corpses.

The narrative of *Slaughterhouse-Five* is largely concerned with the experiences of Billy Pilgrim, an American prisoner of the Germans, Vonnegut's surrogate, who hides in a Dresden slaughterhouse during the firebombing, and, after repatriation, is placed under psychiatric care in a veterans hospital. Billy emerges as a science fiction character "unstuck in time" who is abducted by a flying saucer and taken to the planet Tralfamadore. There, the inhabitants can escape from space-time and, in their "telegraphic schizophrenic" style, offer a shrug-commentary on all deaths with the recurrent phrase "So it goes." The phrase brings playfulness to underlying terror and expresses the Tralfamadorian disbelief in the idea of death.

"So it goes" unifies the diverse filmic flashes that make up the book's sequence as Billy Pilgrim moves back and forth in time and space between his conventional optometry practice in Ilium, New York, wartime Germany, psychiatric hospitals, and the planet Tralfamadore. He is sometimes accompanied by Vonnegut himself, who makes a comment here and there about his own main character. Vonnegut brings an awareness of Hiroshima to *Slaughterhouse-Five*, which he also writes about in other books. He and Billy become our guides in navigating the murderous twentieth century.

Slaughterhouse-Five is about feeling and not feeling,

about remembering and not remembering, about looking and not looking back, about dying and not dying, about living and not living. Vonnegut suggests as "a good epitaph for Billy Pilgrim—and for me too. EVERYTHING WAS BEAUTIFUL AND NOTHING HURT." The tombstone containing the epitaph applies not only to the Vonnegut character but, in Vonnegut's mind, to the rest of us who are not quite alive in our present age of numbing. All this is put forward in Vonnegut's brand of gallows humor, in which a seemingly light touch evokes extreme horror.

A large common theme runs through Camus's insistence on scandalous deaths, Vonnegut's "duty-dance with death" (part of the subtitle of *Slaughterhouse-Five*), and Beckett's life-giving despair, as well as in the work of other survivor-writers and filmmakers, including Tadeusz Borowski's *This Way for the Gas, Ladies and Gentlemen* and the nuclear insanity of Stanley Kubrick's *Dr. Strangelove*. They all tell us that civilization—human life itself—is threatened, dying, or dead: that we must recognize this death or near death, pursue it, record it, enter into it, if we are to learn the truth about ourselves, if we are to go on living as a species.

Covid-19, at least so far, has been creating its own survivor legacy more from a medical than an artistic standpoint. The legacy includes physicians, medics, and epidemiologists who bring new experience, new questions, and sometimes new confusions to the ongoing endeavor.

These patients, healers, and an increasing number of people who become both are bringing valuable forms of witness to the nature and reach of this catastrophic disease.

All these witnesses tell and retell what they have learned. There will undoubtedly emerge creative survivors whose imaginations will do for Covid-19 what Camus, Vonnegut, and others have done for war, for nuclear and climate threats, and for mass killing and dying in general. Such imaginative survivors could provide important models that spread widely and contribute to national and international responses to the Covid catastrophe.

Afterword

Imagining the Real

This book is about survivor power. I have argued that immediate survivors are uniquely capable of confronting and taking in the actuality of a catastrophe, of, in philosopher Martin Buber's term, "imagining the real."

To do that, those immediate survivors become the bearers of catastrophic truth, which is the source of their wisdom. That requires of them an openness not only to pain but also to change. To bring one's imagination to bear on extreme trauma is to undergo a major alteration of the self. That self-alteration can be a step in the direction of healing. The healing process can also affect, and be affected by, more distant survivors of an all-enveloping catastrophe like Covid-19.

That same experience of death and rebirth can be made available to future generations, who may draw upon it from the standpoint of their own struggles and threats.

I have referred to Václav Havel's principle of "living in truth," both experientially and politically. Imagining the real is a way of living the truth of catastrophe. It pertains to each of the survivor struggles I have discussed in this book.

Hibakusha imagined the real when they expanded their Hiroshima experience to worldwide nuclear threat. Survivors in general do so in their struggles to find meaning in catastrophe. They make use of their death anxiety and seek to transcend their apocalyptic images. Witnessing professionals, whether or not survivors themselves, take on the task of exposing and combatting catastrophic threats and bringing that knowledge and advocacy to their society. The mourning process requires facing the reality of loss. And the legacy of survivors to future generations has to do with their providing that original experience and imagination of catastrophic reality.

In all these ways of imagining the real, active survivors emerge from passive victims.

We return to the observation I made in the first chapter of this book: for anyone encountering death there are the alternatives of closing down or opening out. To close down completely is to stay numbed or limit oneself to a sense of victimization. We are able to call forth alternatives that stem from the often unrecognized capacities of the human mind.

One such alternative is what I call the *protean self*, an expression of the self as always in process—as being many-sided rather than monolithic, and resilient rather than fixed.

The protean self is a way of adapting to significant historical dislocation and change. Such dislocation and change are caused by catastrophe, such as the Covid-19 pandemic, war or the threat of war, or the ongoing threats of climate change.

The protean self emerges from dislocation, from the widespread feeling that we are losing our psychological moorings. We feel ourselves buffeted about by unmanageable historical forces and social uncertainties. But rather than collapse under these threats and pulls, the self can instead adapt and prevail. It makes use of bits and pieces here and there and somehow keeps going. What may seem to be mere tactical flexibility, or just bungling along, turns out to be much more than that. We find ourselves evolving a self of many possibilities, one that has risks and pitfalls but at the same time holds out considerable promise for the human future.

We don't just do it alone. Collective proteanism can enable us to remain engaged with trauma and can contribute to the recovery from catastrophe. The alternative can be collective stasis or retreat into cultlike fixity.

We seem to struggle always between proteanism and the

fixity of fundamentalism and cultism. Indeed, fundamentalism and cultism can be a reaction to the anxieties of protean multiplicity and the loss of a sense of stability. That fixity suppresses our symbolizing function and can lead to political totalism or guru-centered efforts at owning reality.

In this way, totalistic behavior interferes with the profound connection between self and history. Proteanism, in contrast, seeks to restore the self's broader symbolizing capacity and its overall connection to the historical process.

Proteanism, though offering no guarantees about the human future, can help us to stem the cultist loss of reality and reassert the imagining of the real.

Proteanism involves choice. But that malleability, if it is to be sustained, requires accompanying elements of stability, or what can be called *grounding*. That grounding can contain not only individual psychological but historical and biological components. At the individual level, the self can include relatively stable elements existing in tandem with areas of change and transformation. There can be a back-and-forth dynamic between these stable elements and protean explorations.

Sigmund Freud and Carl Jung can offer us examples of such grounded proteanism. Lewis Mumford, the humanist and social critic, in a 1964 essay, told how each man in lonely isolation—Freud late at night in his study in Vienna and Jung in his Bollingen Tower—spun out the wildly imaginative ideas that were to have such a profound impact on the twentieth century and beyond. But at the same time, as Mumford pointed out, each of the two men carried on relatively conventional lives as dedicated physicians who met with patients regularly, had a long and stable marriage and family life, and lived at the same residences for decades.

Jung, while recognizing his Bollingen experience as explorations in psychosis, emphasized that "my family and my profession remained the base to which I could always return, assuring me that I was an actually existing, ordinary person." Mumford pointed out that in these commitments as family men, teachers, and physicians, Freud and Jung "kept their hold on reality." That anchoring enabled them to lead something close to a double life, in which the very orderliness and stability of their demanding routines, rather than conflicting with their expression of bold imagination, could well have made that expression possible. The stable components in their lives enabled both men to cope with the catastrophe of

World War I and the uneasy survival of the psychoanalytic movement.*

The same was true for Havel in his remarkable merger of
proteanism and groundedness. He spoke of a "new experience of being, a renewed rootedness in the universe, a
newly grasped sense of 'higher responsibility' . . . to the
human community." And a "'human order,' which no
political order can replace." All this required rejecting the
lies of oppressors in favor of imagining the real.

Such grounded proteanism can provide a path for our
species. That is, proteanism presses toward human commonality, as opposed to the fixed and absolute moral and
psychological divisions favored by fundamentalism. For
there is a trajectory, never automatic but always possible,
from the protean self to the species self—to the formation
of a sense of self based significantly upon one's connection to humankind. Proteanism provides no panacea for
catastrophe; what it does offer is a potential for change

---

* I do not discuss here Jung's controversial relationship to World War II,
during which he apparently had some attraction to the Nazis and served
as editor of a journal they controlled.

and renewal, for tapping human resilience. In any case, proteanism is integral to our historical situation, to our contemporary fate.

Catastrophe calls on us to bring the mind to bear upon the most unpalatable truths of our historical epoch, to expand the limits of imagination on behalf of survival. The task is not easy. What is required of us is not only calling forth end-of-the-world imagery but in some degree mastering it, giving it a place in our aesthetic and moral narratives.

It is futile to try to dismiss images of Hiroshima and Auschwitz—or of nuclear threat, climate change, and Covid-19—from human consciousness, as so many groups and individuals try to do. That misguided effort deprives us of our current truths as well as our history—of what and where we have been—and thereby impedes our efforts to alter collective behavior.

We need to confront whatever catastrophe we experience and recognize its interaction with everyday life. Only in that way can we deepen and facilitate our imagination as it struggles with such daunting contemporary issues as the destruction of democracy, racism, and Covid-19.

What we speak of as future renewal is inseparable from present engagement. That engagement is built on survivor energies and involves witnessing professionals, political leaders, and ordinary citizens.

Acknowledgments

Nancy Rosenblum's ideas enriched the book. Much more than that, she has deeply enriched the life of its author. Jane Isay, as always, did important editing. I have been in active dialogue with friends and colleagues including Peter Balakian, James Carroll, Cathy Caruth, Judith Herman, and Charles Strozier.

Bailey Georges contributed suggestions for the text, invaluable editing, and overall coordination.

Richard Morris, my agent, offered constant counsel and good advice. Carolyn Mugar provided research support and great encouragement. Ellen Adler and Jay Gupta at The New Press did much to improve the manuscript and to connect it to prevailing social currents. Managing editor Maury Botton and copyeditor Eileen G. Chetti helped turn the manuscript into a book.

Notes

1: Catastrophe and Survivors

4 Definitions of "survivor" and "victim" from the Merriam-Webster Dictionary and the Oxford English Dictionary.

2: The Prophetic Survivors of Hiroshima

14 Much of this chapter is drawn from: Robert Jay Lifton, *Death in Life: Survivors of Hiroshima* (Chapel Hill: University of North Carolina Press [1968], 1991).

14 "twisted iron hospital bed": Michihiko Hachiya, *Hiroshima Diary*, trans. and ed. Warner Wells (Chapel Hill: University of North Carolina Press, 1955), 31.

14 "a fearful silence": Yōko Ōta, *Shikabane no Machi* (Town of Corpses) (Tokyo: Kawade Shobo, 1955), 63.

20 Hidankyo: See Nihon Hidankyo, "Message to the World," www
.ne.jp/asahi/hidankyo/nihon/english/about/about1-02.html, and "Atomic
Bomb Victims Appeal," www.ne.jp/asahi/hidankyo/nihon/english/about
/about3-02.html.

3: The Struggle for Meaning

27 Chaim Kaplan diary: See Chaim Kaplan, "A Journal of the Warsaw
Ghetto," *Commentary*, November, 1965, 42-58.

29 the example of Primo Levi: There has been controversy about the
details of his death, whether as an accident or suicide. For a contrasting
view, see Diego Gambetta, "Primo Levi's Last Moments," *Boston Review*,
June 1, 1999.

36 Patients in psychotherapy: Descriptions of patients are from the psy-
chotherapeutic practice of Charles B. Strozier. See Robert Jay Lifton and
Charles B. Strozier, "The Psychological Pandemic: Can We Confront Our
Death Anxiety?," *Bulletin of the Atomic Scientists*, March 1, 2021.

40 "numbing litany of bad news": Indrajit Samarajiva, "I Lived Through
Collapse. America Is Already There," *GEN Medium*, September 26, 2020.

4: Rejecting Catastrophe and Survival

46 support a fast track: Yasmeen Abutaleb, Laurie McGinley, and
Carolyn Y. Johnson, "How the 'Deep State' Scientists Vilified by Trump
Helped Him Deliver an Unprecedented Achievement," *Washington Post*,
December 14, 2020.

46 "miraculously goes away": Alyson Hurt, Tamara Keith and Audrey
Carlsen, "Timeline: What Trump Has Said and Done About the Coronavirus," National Public Radio, April 21, 2020.

50 Lost Cause . . . American Civil War: See David W. Blight, "Lost Cause," *Encyclopedia Britannica*, September 20, 2021.

51 "the fury that had been rising" and "Lost Cause theologians": Susan Neiman, *Learning from the Germans: Race and the Memory of Evil* (New York: Farrar, Straus and Giroux, 2019), 180, 188.

53 Todd Gitlin calls the "Vortex": Todd Gitlin, "Flat Earthers and Feedback Loops," *BillMoyers.com*, August 1, 2017.

54 a perversive immoralism: Robert Jay Lifton and Nancy Rosenblum, "Donald Trump, the Immoralist," *New York Daily News*, August 31, 2020.

58 "most incendiary": See Barbara Walter interviewed by Lindsay Morgan on the *Talking Policy* podcast episode "Is the U.S. Headed Toward Civil War?," *University of California Institute on Global Conflict and Cooperation,* January 3, 2022.

59 "health misinformation": Sam Schechner, Jeff Horwitz, and Emily Glazer "How Facebook Hobbled Mark Zuckerberg's Bid to Get America Vaccinated," *Wall Street Journal*, September 17, 2021.

59 "attention economy": Michael H. Goldhaber, "Attention Shoppers!," *Wired*, December 1, 1997.

59 "you have power": Michael Goldhaber interviewed by Charlie Warzel, "I Talked to the Cassandra of the Internet Age," *New York Times*, February 4, 2021.

60 "living in truth": See Václav Havel, "The Power of the Powerless," in *Living in Truth* (London: Faber and Faber, 1987).

60 enacting democracy: See Nancy L. Rosenblum and Russell Muirhead, *A Lot of People Are Saying: The New Conspiracism and the Assault on Democracy* (New Jersey: Princeton University Press, 2019), 14, 158–165.

5: The Mourning Paradox

66 "we *feel lost* ourselves": Kathleen Woodward, "Freud and Barthes: Theorizing Mourning, Sustaining Grief," *Discourse* 13, no. 1 (1990): 93.

66 The Mitscherlichs: Alexander and Margarete Mitscherlich, *Inability to Mourn: Principles of Collective Behavior* (New York: Grove Press, [1975] 1984).

69 My Lai massacre: My interviews with the American My Lai survivor in *Home from the War: Vietnam Veterans—Neither Victims Nor Executioners* (New York: Simon & Schuster, 1973). And Martin Gershen, *Destroy or Die: The True Story of Mylai* (New Rochelle, NY: Arlington House, 1971).

72 threw their medals back: Lifton, *Home from the War*, 178.

74 "the foulness of death": See references in Robert Jay Lifton, *The Broken Connection: On Death and the Continuity of Life* (New York: Simon & Schuster, 1979), 93.

75 "An anonymous mass": Primo Levi, *Survival in Auschwitz: The Nazi Assault on Humanity* (New York: Collier, 1961), 82.

76 "No Hint of National Mourning": Micki McElya, "Almost 90,000 Dead and No Hint of National Mourning. Are These Deaths Not 'Ours'?," *Washington Post*, May 15, 2020.

82 "humanity behind the statistics": Cleve Jones, "How One Man's Idea for the AIDS Quilt Made the Country Pay Attention," *Washington Post*, October 9, 2016.

83 "fire burning in their hearts": Alex Seitz-Wald, "What Would a Covid Memorial Look Like? Designers Share Ideas for 'Unprecedented' Tribute," *NBC News*, October 11, 2021.

83 "we owe it to the million": Carlie Porterfield, "Inside the Movement to Build a National Covid Memorial," *Forbes*, March 18, 2022.

6: Activist Witnessing

87 "a vast grass-roots": Sheryl Gay Stolberg, "Scarred by Covid, Survivors and Victims' Families Aim to Be a Political Force," *New York Times*, July 20, 2021.

94 "a giant fireball": Eugene Rabinowitch, "Five Years After," in *The Atomic Age,* ed. Morton Grodzins and Eugene Rabinowitch (New York: Basic Books, 1963), 156.

102 "step down . . . speak out": Irwin Redlener, "It's Time for Trump's Top Doctors to Step Down and Speak Up," *Daily Beast*, October 15, 2020.

103 Fauci rejected: Anthony S. Fauci interviewed by Donald G. McNeil Jr., "Fauci on What Working for Trump Was Really Like," *New York Times,* January 24, 2021.

7: The Legacy of Survivors

107 Definitions of "legacy" from the Merriam-Webster Dictionary and the Oxford English Dictionary.

107 "the concept of the generation": José Ortega y Gasset, *What Is Philosophy?* (New York: W.W. Norton & Company, 1960), 33–34.

113 Pinchas Gutter quotations are from conversations with Gutter through the Dimensions in Testimony project, https://iwitness.usc.edu/dit /pinchas.

115 British social scientist: Ed Prideaux, "How to Heal the 'Mass Trauma' of Covid-19," BBC, February 3, 2021.

115 "The Artist carries death": Heinrich Böll, *The Clown*, trans. Leila Vennewitz (Brooklyn, NY: Melville House, [1963] 2010).

116 "as a scandal": Germaine Brée, *Camus* (New Brunswick, NJ: Rutgers University Press, 1959).

116 "no death reverberated": Albert Camus, *Œuvres complètes vol. 2*, eds. Jacqueline Lévi-Valensi, Raymond Gay-Crosier et al. (Paris: Gallimard, 2006–8), 710.

117 "What had to be done": Albert Camus, *The Plague* (New York: Alfred A. Knopf, 1948), 308.

118 "so short and jumbled": Kurt Vonnegut, *Slaughterhouse-Five, or The Children's Crusade: A Duty-Dance with Death* (New York: Delacorte Press, 1969), 17.

Afterword: Imagining the Real

128 Lewis Mumford, the humanist: Lewis Mumford, "Who Invented the Demons?," *New Yorker*, May 23, 1964, 155–85.

130 "new experience of being": Havel, *Living in Truth*, 118.

INDEX

INDEX

About the Author

Robert Jay Lifton is an American psychiatrist and author whose subjects have been holocaust, mass violence, and renewal in the twentieth and twenty-first centuries. His books include such seminal works as the National Book Award–winning *Death in Life: Survivors of Hiroshima,* the *Los Angeles Times* Book Prize–winning *The Nazi Doctors*, the National Book Award–nominated *Home from the War: Vietnam Veterans—Neither Victims Nor Executioners,* as well as *The Climate Swerve* and *Losing Reality* (both from The New Press). He has taught at Yale University, Harvard University, and the City University of New York. He lives in New York City and Massachusetts.

Publishing in the Public Interest

Thank you for reading this book published by The New Press; we hope you enjoyed it. New Press books and authors play a crucial role in sparking conversations about the key political and social issues of our day.

We hope that you will stay in touch with us. Here are a few ways to keep up to date with our books, events, and the issues we cover:

- Sign up at www.thenewpress.com/subscribe to receive updates on New Press authors and issues and to be notified about local events
- www.facebook.com/newpressbooks
- www.twitter.com/thenewpress
- www.instagram.com/thenewpress

Please consider buying New Press books not only for yourself, but also for friends and family and to donate to schools, libraries, community centers, prison libraries, and other organizations involved with the issues our authors write about.

The New Press is a 501(c)(3) nonprofit organization; if you wish to support our work with a tax-deductible gift please visit www.thenewpress.com/donate or use the QR code below.